6/18

HEALING WITH
HEMP
CBD OIL

Other Square One Titles by Earl Mindell

The Happiness Effect

What You Must Know About Allergy Relief
with Pamela Wartian Smith, MD, MPH

What You Must Know About Homeopathic Remedies

HEALING WITH
HEMP
CBD OIL

A SIMPLE GUIDE TO USING POWERFUL AND PROVEN HEALTH BENEFITS OF CBD

Earl Mindell, RPh, MH, PhD

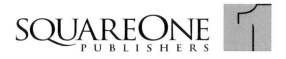

SQUAREONE
PUBLISHERS

The information and advice contained in this book are based upon the research and the personal and professional experiences of the authors. They are not intended as a substitute for consulting with a health care professional. The publisher and author are not responsible for any adverse effects or consequences resulting from the use of any of the suggestions, preparations, or procedures discussed in this book. All matters pertaining to your physical health should be supervised by a health care professional. It is a sign of wisdom, not cowardice, to seek a second or third opinion.

EDITOR: Erica Shur
COVER DESIGNER: Jeannie Tudor
TYPESETTER: Gary A. Rosenberg (InDesign)

Square One Publishers
115 Herricks Road
Garden City Park, NY 11040
(516) 535-2010 • (877) 900-BOOK
www.squareonepublishers.com

Library of Congress Cataloging-in-Publication Data
Names: Mindell, Earl, author.
Title: Healing with hemp CBD oil : a simple guide to using powerful and
   proven health benefits of CBD / Earl Mindell, RPh, PhD.
Description: Garden City Park, NY : Square One Publishers, [2018] | Includes
   bibliographical references and index.
Identifiers: LCCN 2017042197 (print) | LCCN 2017039200 (ebook) | ISBN
   9780757004551 (paperback) | ISBN 9780757054556
Subjects: LCSH: Cannabis—Therapeutic use. | Hemp seed oil—Therapeutic use.
   | Hemp—Therapeutic use.
Classification: LCC RM666.C266 M56 2017 (ebook) | LCC RM666.C266 (print) |
   DDC 615.7/827—dc23
LC record available at HYPERLINK "https://lccn.loc.gov/2017042197" https://lccn.loc.
gov/2017042197

Printed in the United States of America

10   9   8   7   6   5   4   3   2

Contents

To my wife and soulmate, Gail,
to our children, Alanna and Evan,
and to our grandchildren,
Lily and Ryan.

Acknowledgments

I wish to express my deep and lasting appreciation to my friends, associates and especially to my family, Gail, Alanna, Evan, Lily and Ryan, for their assistance and understanding in the preparation of this book.

I would like to thank my editors at Square One, Erica Shur and Caroline Smith, for all their talent and efforts in making sure that all the material in this work was clear and accessible.

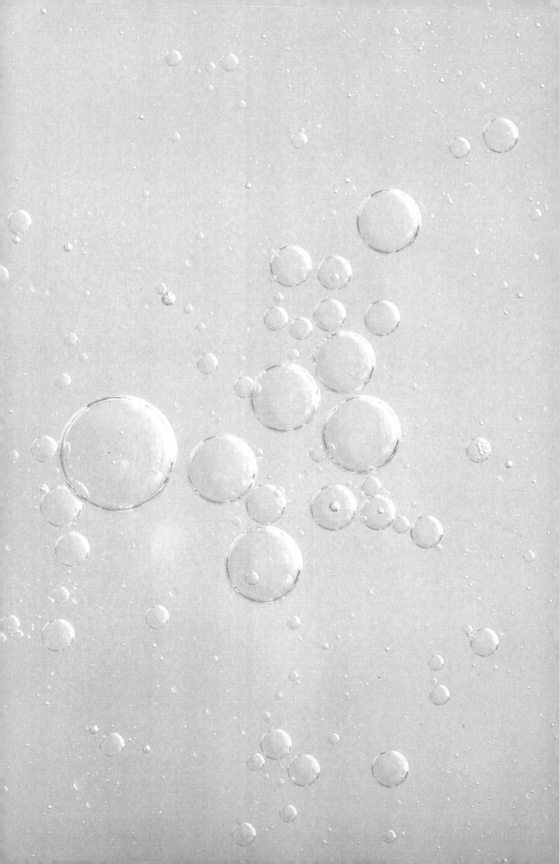

Introduction

Imagine that researchers had found a naturally occurring substance that could effectively overcome dozens of health disorders without any serious side effects. Now imagine that the plant in which this substance was found had been banned in this country because, as a commercially grown crop, it threatened other competing "cash" crops. As new studies showed its many medical benefits, our laws continued to prevent farmers from planting an easy-to-grow crop that requires few, if any, pesticides or herbicides. If you think that sounds so crazy that it couldn't be true, think again. For the last seventy years, the Federal government has prohibited farmers from commercially growing the hemp plant. In doing so, it has effectively prevented American companies from making available hemp extracts with CBD—the very compound that science has found to be an amazing and versatile healer.

As it turns out, hemp is a relative of marijuana. Both are *cannabis* plants, as are many other plants. However, while marijuana is high in THC, the chemical compound that accounts for marijuana's psychoactive effects, hemp contains too little of this chemical to get anyone high. On the other hand, while the majority of available marijuana contains a relatively low level of the healing compound CBD, hemp is high in CBD—which has no psychoactive effects and is non-toxicating. Yet as you will discover in the chapters that follow, for decades, the hemp plant has been outlawed along with marijuana because the government has falsely classified it as a dangerous Schedule 1 drug. And while more and more states are legalizing the growth and sale of marijuana, hemp is still not permitted to be grown as a commercial crop.

As a registered pharmacist, I have witnessed the amazing growth of pharmaceutical companies over the years. I have also seen too many of these companies produce drugs that may relieve specific symptoms, but come with dangerous side effects. I have always looked for natural products that can provide the same relief without the risk of side effects. That is not to say that pharmaceutical companies don't produce life-saving drugs, because they do.

However, nature has provided us with many alternative solutions that work well. Over the years, as I read more about the many benefits of hemp oil extracts and CBD, I discovered that hemp's classification as a Schedule 1 drug made no sense in light of the available scientific research. I needed to know more.

Healing With Hemp CBD Oil is the result of my investigation into this important product. The book is divided into two parts. Part One presents the basics of hemp. It begins with a look at hemp's impressive history and its importance as a popular crop grown throughout the world. It goes on to explain the groundbreaking scientific research into hemp oil and its healing effects on the body. Because of the amount of misinformation about hemp oil products, Chapter 4 is devoted to making you a smart consumer who knows how to buy, use, and store hemp oil-based products. Part One concludes with an eye-opening review of the law, medicine, and CBD.

Part Two provides an A-to-Z listing of specific health disorders and how hemp oil can be used to relieve them. Each entry includes an explanation of the problem, its most common symptoms, its causes, and its standard conventional treatment and side effects, if any. The entry concludes with a discussion of how you can use hemp oil to improve your health. At the end of the book, a resource section guides you to the organizations and websites that can assist you in learning more about hemp. For those who wish to read the research papers and articles on which this book was based, you'll also find an extensive list of references.

The information presented in this book is not meant to replace the medical advice given to you by your physician. It is designed to provide the facts you need to know to make informed decisions about your health. If in reading this book you find a treatment that is of interest to you, do not be afraid to discuss it with your doctor. You can play an important role in your own health or healing process.

As much as I want to guide you to safe treatments for your health problems, I also want this book to get you angry. The United States government has banned our farmers from commercially growing hemp, one of the world's most important crops. After reading the pages that follow, I hope you agree that the time has come to change the law and allow both our farmers and our people to benefit from this amazing plant.

PART ONE

Hemp Oil and CBD Basics

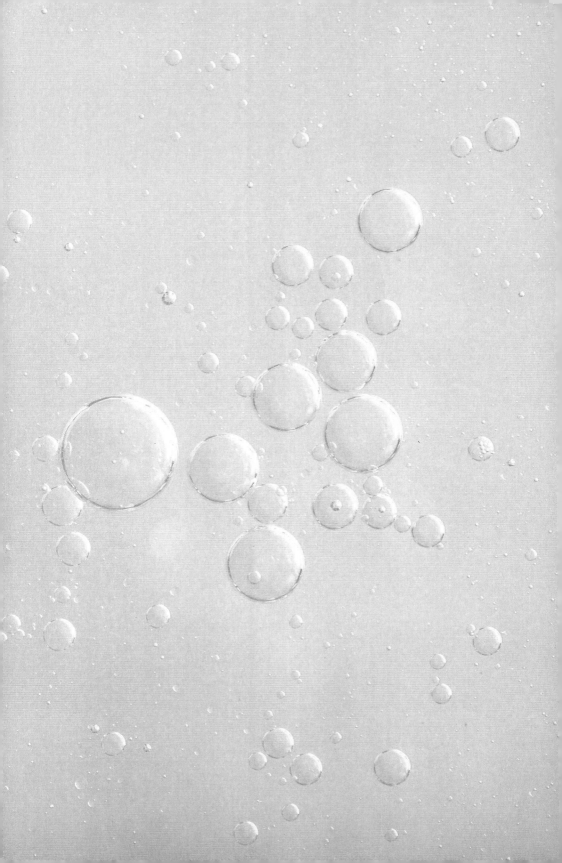

1.

The History of Hemp

emp's history spans several thousand years; it was one of the first plants to be grown for purposes other than food. It had multiple uses in ancient Chinese and Indian cultures, ranging from a religious symbol to a tonic to a foundation for industrial materials. Centuries later, hemp spread to the Western world, where America's Founding Fathers used paper made from hemp fibers to draft the most important documents of our civilization. The United States government officially noted the medicinal qualities of hemp and cannabis in 1850, although the unique benefits of cannabidiol (CBD) and delta-9-tetrahydrocannabinol (THC)—the two major components of the plants' chemical make-ups—wouldn't be specified until the 1960s.

If hemp was such an essential component of societies around the world, why then was its cultivation banned in the United States in the 1900s? If CBD is a non-intoxicating "decaffeinated" version of THC—why are they looped together as one and the same in our laws? You may be surprised to learn that all it took to make the public fearful of cannabis and hemp were the narrow-minded agendas of powerful politicians and industry leaders. As you will see, they succeeded in attaching a stigma to these plants that even science, history, and countless success stories have failed to eradicate. In this chapter, we do our part to dispel that stigma by exploring the fascinating history of the hemp plant and its prominent compound, CBD.

HEMP'S RISE AND FALL

Hemp has been grown all over the world for at least 12,000 years. It is a variety of the *Cannabis Sativa L.* plant—a term most people associate with its close relative, marijuana. Hemp differs from marijuana, however, in that it lacks a substantial amount of THC, the chemical responsible for its cousin's psychoactive properties. True food and fiber varieties of hemp are naturally low in THC and are significantly high in CBD. These plants have completely different DNA from drug varieties of marijuana and are the ideal source for CBD. As a commercial crop, hemp has also proven its value in so many ways—producing fabric, fibers, lotions, soaps, cooking oil, and fuel, as well as nutritional supplements. In fact, it is estimated that hemp has over an astounding 25,000 unique uses. As you read on, you will learn why this highly versatile plant has suffered from stigma despite its intrinsic industrial, agricultural and medical value.

Hemp Throughout the Ages

Forms of the cannabis plant, including hemp, have been promoted as medicine since ancient times. One of the earliest mentions of hemp as a medicine was in a pharmacopeia—a book of remedies—called the *Shen-nung Pen-ts'ao Ching*. This book is thought to be the world's oldest medicinal guide. It was based on traditional Chinese treatments passed down from the time of the emperor Shen Nung, who lived around 2700 BC. The complete guide itself, however, was not compiled until the first or second century AD. The Chinese also created the first piece of paper completely made from hemp by 150 BC. Some of the oldest known writings, such as Buddhist texts from 100–200 AD, were scribed on hemp paper.

The Persian prophet Zoroaster placed hemp at the topmost rank in the *Zend-Avesta*, a list of over 10,000 medicinal plants written in approximately 1000 B.C. In ancient Indian culture, written and oral tradition states that the god Indra's favorite drink was made of hemp, while the Buddha Siddhartha ate only hemp and its seeds for years. The sacred Indian text *Atharva Veda*, written around 1400 BC, listed cannabis as a remedy for distress. It also described the throwing of hemp boughs into a fire as a magical ritual that fought evil forces. Ancient Greek physician Hippocrates (460-370 BC)—whose teachings are still observed in Western medicine today—recommended the use of cannabis in various treatments.

Hemp likely spread to Europe around 1200 BC, although it was not a prevalent crop until the start of the Middle Ages, around 500 AD. It became significant to the European economy mostly in the manufacture of sails and ropes. Italy, especially, was a hub for hemp production. The Italians prided themselves on their superior ships and fine clothing made of hemp. A factory called the Tana was built in Venice to enforce high standards for hemp quality and durability. In the 1500s, realizing the success that Italy and the rest of Europe had enjoyed, England entered the hemp market. King Henry VIII imposed a fine on farmers who did not dedicate at least a quarter-acre of their land to hemp cultivation. Farmers, however, were hesitant to comply because they did not profit from hemp as much as they did from grains or other crops. As a result, England imported most of its hemp from Russia—the largest source and exporter of hemp in the 1600s.

Hemp had reached America by the sixteenth century, and its versatility and valuable roles were well-known. In 1619, the First General Assembly of Virginia established a law requiring farmers to grow hemp: "For hemp also . . . we do require and enjoin all householders of this colony, that have any of those seeds, to make trial thereof the next season." Hemp was vital in manufacturing the sailboat canvasses and ropes needed for transportation, trade, and navies in America and around the world. It was even used as a form of currency in tax payments.

Many of the Founding Fathers grew their own hemp. For example, George Washington often wrote about the hemp crop being grown at all five of his farms. Initially, he seemed concerned about its potential profitability and whether the hemp would thrive on American soil, as he wrote in a 1765 letter: ". . . as they [hemp and flax] are articles altogether new to us . . . I believe not much of our lands well adapted for them." By 1794, these worries were quashed, as Washington wrote to his farm manager: "I am very glad to hear that the gardener has saved so much . . . of the India Hemp . . . the Hemp may be sown anywhere."

Thomas Jefferson printed the first two drafts of the Declaration of Independence on hemp paper, although the final copy was eventually printed on parchment. Benjamin Franklin published many articles about hemp in the newspaper he printed, the *Pennsylvania Gazette*. One such article, which can now be found in the Gilder Lehrman Institute of American History, reproduced an entry from Ephraim Chambers's *Universal Dictionary*. The entry described how to grow hemp and what its benefits were: "The Seed is said to have the Faculty of abating Venereal desires . . . and the Leaves are held good against Burns. . . . The Culture and Management of Hemp, makes a considerable Article in Agriculture." And while it is rumored that Betsy Ross used hemp cloth to sew together the first American flag, it is a fact that many of the early American flags were made of hemp material. Hemp fiber continued to be widely used in paper until the nineteenth century, when the woodpulping process, the timber industry, and the factory production of paper became more prominent.

In 1839, a surgeon named William Brooke O'Shaughnessy brought cannabis into mainstream medicine after learning of its medical benefits in India, and by 1850, it was added to the US Pharmacopeia list of Medicines and Dietary Supplements. Less than a century later, the plant would be outlawed—despite its long history and its importance as one of the backbones of American culture. What happened? How did cannabis and hemp experience such a large fall from grace, and how come laws re-allowing hemp cultivation have only recently started to gain traction? We will explore these questions in the next section.

Why Was Hemp Banned?

As you can see, for centuries, hemp enjoyed universal endorsement. But in the first half of the twentieth century, things began to change. In 1906, Congress passed the Pure Food and Drug Act. This Act established the Food and Drug Administration (FDA) and required food labels to be accurate and honest. Under this Act, ten ingredients including cannabis were deemed "addictive." While not outlawed, these ingredients were required to be clearly labeled on food and medical products. Backlash against cannabis and hemp emerged around this time. During the turmoil of the Mexican Revolution (1910–1920), immigrants from Mexico introduced the recreational use of cannabis to the United States.

Although Americans had already been using drugs recreationally in opium and hashish parlors, the immigrants became the face of drug use. Newspapers told stories of crimes committed by people under the influence of drugs. Racist officials started grouping cannabis and hemp together under the same name "marijuana," a Mexican slang term, to associate the plants with something foreign and dangerous. The American people seemed unaware that this "marijuana" was the same cannabis and hemp they had been cultivating and using for years.

By the 1930s, all states had regulations against marijuana and the Federal Bureau of Narcotics (FBN) had been established. The FBN proposed to replace the Harrison Narcotics Tax Act, which was established in 1914 with the Uniform State Narcotic Drug Act of 1934. This Act was created in response to the public demand for a uniform, nationwide law regarding illegal drugs. It mostly concerned opiates and cocaine, but noted that if any state wished to regulate marijuana, the law could be applied. These so-called "poisons" could be seized by the authorities if citizens were found to be in possession.

The FBN sought to ban all recreational drugs. Its commissioner, Harry Anslinger, was very vocal in his belief that cannabis caused people to become aggressive and deviant. Propaganda films and advertisements were produced, associating cannabis and hemp with getting high, laziness, violence, and "reefer madness"—even though hemp does not contain any significant amount of the psychoactive and intoxicating THC element.

Racism, Fear, and Marijuana

The hysteria surrounding cannabis and hemp was based on racist ideas. Mexicans were not the only target; marijuana was also linked with black people and "viciousness." Harry Anslinger promoted a campaign against black jazz musicians, such as Louis Armstrong and Duke Ellington, by stating that their "Satanic" music was created through the use of marijuana, and that this music—and the dancing that accompanied it—made white women become sexual and unruly. To pinpoint his line of attack, Anslinger wrote to his agents, "Please prepare all cases in your jurisdiction involving musicians in violation of marijuana laws. We will have a great national round-up arrest of all such persons on a single day." He later clarified that this raid would affect not "the good musicians, but the jazz type," and that "the increase [in drug addiction] is practically 100 percent among [black] people." Anslinger and the FBN's relentless pursuit of marijuana holders was a vendetta backed not by scientific research, but by personal biases.

Meanwhile, William Randolph Hearst, founder of media corporation Hearst, led a movement against hemp for years through yellow journalism—exaggerated, attention-grabbing news that was never backed up with reliable research. His newspapers painted the picture of marijuana as a drug smoked by lazy, violent Mexican people. Like Harry Anslinger, Hearst also likely held a racist vendetta: According to the *Smithsonian Magazine,* Hearst controlled over a half-million acres of land in Mexico that was pillaged by the Mexican General Pancho Villa. The frightening propaganda and advertisements, promoted by the government and influential people like Anslinger and Hearst, was successful. The American public became fearful of marijuana, and wary of hemp by association.

Economics may have also played a role in the demonization of cannabis. In his 1973 book, *The Emperor Wears No Clothes,* Jack Herer suggests that certain industries may have felt threatened by hemp production. Such industries may have included timber, because of hemp's popularity in paper products, and nylon, which at the time was a new, synthetic fabric that was competing with hemp textiles. Manufacturers of these products sought to kill the competition by drawing comparisons between hemp and its relative, marijuana.

Because fabric made from hemp is long lasting and is naturally pest-resistant (i.e., its production does not require the heavy use of chemical pesticides), its success may have been perceived as a threat to the cotton industry as well. The production of cotton accounts for nearly half of the chemical pesticide use in the United States. A counter argument to this theory was presented in a 2014 investigation by Brian Dunning with skeptoid.com, who argued against the urban legend that William Randolph Hearst conspired to make hemp illegal in the United States. While this theory has been met with some controversy, there is no question that by creating a negative perception of hemp in the public's mind, these industries would reap the benefits of weakening their competition.

The Marijuana Tax Act

In 1937, the Marijuana Tax Act was passed, which enforced a tax on the sale of cannabis. If you were found to be in possession of cannabis without having paid a federal revenue tax, or failed to register the plants with the Federal Bureau of Narcotics, you would be subject to arrest. The law also affected doctors and pharmacists who prescribed cannabis, as they had to go through an arduous process to attain it and paid a special tax for prescribing it. If they too did not follow these procedures, they were prone to hefty fines, imprisonment, or both. At this time, the American Medical Association was strongly opposed to outlawing marijuana and did not see it as the addictive drug that it was painted to be, stating:

> There is positively no evidence to indicate the abuse of cannabis as a medicinal agent or to show that its medicinal use is leading to the development of cannabis addiction. Cannabis at the present time is slightly used for medicinal purposes, but it would seem worthwhile to maintain its status as a medicinal agent for such purposes as it now has. There is a possibility that a restudy of the drug by modern means may show other advantages to be derived from its medicinal use.

Eventually, the Marijuana Tax Act was ruled unconstitutional after the 1969 court case *Leary v. United States*. In 1965, a Harvard professor named Dr. Timothy Leary had been arrested in Texas as he was returning from a vacation in Mexico. Although a small amount of marijuana was found in his daughter's clothing, he took responsibility for its possession in violation of the Marijuana Tax Act. While he was initially found guilty and sentenced to thirty years in prison, all charges were dropped under appeal. In 1968, he was arrested once again in California for possession of two marijuana "roaches," and convicted under the same law. When the case was eventually brought to the Supreme Court, the Marijuana Tax Act was found unconstitutional because it violated the Fifth Amendment against self-incrimination. Leary's California conviction was overturned.

The Marijuana Tax Act was replaced by the Comprehensive Drug Abuse and Prevention Control Act in 1970. Title II of this act was the Controlled Substance Act (CSA), which divided drugs into five schedules based on their addictiveness and/or accepted medical use. According to the CSA, hemp and marijuana were listed as "Schedule I Drugs," subsequently prohibiting their consumption and possession. Hemp and marijuana were considered the same, despite hemp's near non-existent THC concentration and lack of psychoactive and intoxicating effects. According to the law, these drugs have "a high potential for abuse" and "no currently accepted medical use in treatment in the United States." The Act made it illegal to grow hemp without a permit, as well. Today, hemp is still being imported from other countries, but a "zero tolerance" level was established, meaning imported hemp products cannot contain more than trace amounts of naturally-occurring THC. The CSA defined "zero" THC as having less than 0.3%. Products with less than 0.3% THC are exempt from the CSA and legal to sell within the US. For example, since sterilized hemp seeds and products that are made from sterilized seeds, textiles, and cosmetics do not have THC, they are allowed to be imported and sold in the United States.

True hemp, meaning certified non-drug varieties of agricultural hemp and their extracts, which contain a full spectrum of naturally occurring phytocannabinoids, are also lawfully imported. When handled properly, these extracts can provide a safe, effective, and sustainable source of CBD.

The Modern-Day Laws

Confusion has arisen because some modern-day state laws and the federal law contradict each other. Cannabis possession is still outlawed at the federal level, but as of 2018, more than thirty states have decriminalized or legalized it at the state level. The Federal government has the authority to punish cannabis possessors even in a state where it is legal, although it is rare that this happens.

Hemp cultivation, meanwhile, still hangs in limbo. The 2014 United States Farm Bill, which determines the country's agricultural and food policies, allows "industrial hemp"—hemp with a THC level below 0.3 percent—to be cultivated for research purposes. The cultivation sites must be certified and registered with the state. Over two dozen states allow farmers to grow industrial hemp for these purposes. In 2015, the Industrial Hemp Farming Act was introduced in Congress. If passed, it would remove all restrictions on cultivating industrial hemp. It would also remove hemp from the list of Schedule I drugs, as long as it has a THC level lower than 0.3 percent. However, this law has yet to be voted through, and is currently in its seventh iteration in the House. Many other laws have also been introduced to free hemp from the same restrictions as a high THC strain of cannabis. These laws aim to differentiate between higher risk cannabis with greater levels of THC and low-to-no risk agricultural hemp, which is non-intoxicating.

A great analogy would be to compare the difference between decaffeinated and regular caffeinated coffee to that of hemp and marijuana. Hemp and hemp-derived CBD products are considered by some to be non-intoxicating versions, or "decaffeinated" alternatives, to marijuana's intoxicating or "caffeinated" products.

In Chapter 3, we will go more in depth into the laws surrounding hemp, marijuana, and CBD.

THE DISCOVERY OF CBD

Although cannabis as a whole has been used as a medication for thousands of years, it has only been in the last century or so that cannabidiol, or CBD, has been extracted from the plant and used on its own to treat medical conditions. In the following sections, we will reveal when and how CBD was first discovered, as well as the significance of its discovery. We will track its history as a supplement and discuss the research that is proving it to be a force of nature.

Initial Research

One of the first known isolations of CBD from the cannabis plant took place in 1940. The findings were detailed in an article in the *Journal of the American Chemical Society* that year. The researchers noted that CBD had "none of the physiological activity typical of marihuana [sic]." Simply put, CBD was

CBD Composition

CBD is made of the chemical elements carbon, hydrogen, and oxygen. Its molecular formula is $C_{21}H_{30}O_2$. THC is made up of the same elements and has the exact same molecular formula; however, the arrangement of the atoms is unique to each compound, so they act in different ways. This variance is what gives THC its psychoactive effects, which CBD does not have. CBD actually counteracts THC's psychoactive effects. An illustration of the different arrangements of THC and CBD can be found in Figure 1.1 below.

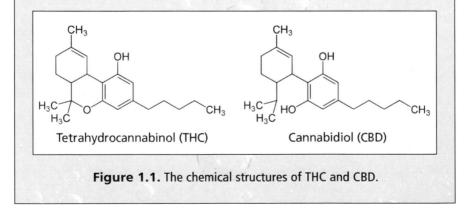

Tetrahydrocannabinol (THC)   Cannabidiol (CBD)

Figure 1.1. The chemical structures of THC and CBD.

found to be nonpsychoactive, meaning that, unlike THC, it does not produce the "high" that is typically associated with cannabis use.

For about twenty years after that initial isolation, research on CBD was limited. But in the early 1960s, a chemist named Dr. Raphael Mechoulam and his group of researchers determined the exact chemical structures of both CBD and THC. (See inset "CBD Composition" on page 12.) Discovering the chemical structure of CBD paved the way for future scientists to understand the nature of CBD and other chemical structures present in cannabis, known as cannabinoids. This is because Dr. Mechoulam's lab discovered that cannabinoids bind to specific receptors inside the body, contrary to the popular belief at the time that they "nonspecifically" altered the structure of cell membranes. Some of the cannabinoid receptors are found in immune system cells, which suggests that cannabinoids may contribute to enhanced immunity.

For over forty years, Dr. Mechoulam continued to study CBD and its effects on conditions such as epilepsy and nausea. He also discovered much about the way CBD acts once it is inside the body. According to an article in the journal *O'Shaughnessy's*, CBD binds to cannabinoid receptors found throughout the peripheral nervous system. Its structure "enables it to get into places in the brain that conventional neurotransmitters cannot reach." It also blocks some kinds of inhibitory neurotransmitters while activating receptors of helpful neurotransmitters, such as serotonin, a mood regulator. You will learn more about the body's response to cannabinoids in Chapter 2.

Recent Interest in Medical Marijuana and CBD

For many years, the THC-dominant strain of marijuana was the most prominent in the United States. Most marijuana consumers were primarily seeking a "high," and growers and dealers catered to them. Because of this selective breeding, the CBD content of cannabis decreased. CBD-dominant strains were practically unheard of in the United States until recently.

Beginning in the 1990s, interest and progress in the medical marijuana movement began to surge. With more benefits of CBD being uncovered every day, even pharmaceutical companies are looking to cash into the business. In 1996, California passed Proposition 215, also known as the Compassionate Use Act. This was the first state-level medical marijuana initiative passed in the country. It allowed patients and their designated caregivers to possess and cultivate marijuana for personal medical use as long as they had a valid doctor's recommendation. Soon, other medical and recreational marijuana initiatives were passed in dozens of other states.

Internationally, a British company called GW Pharmaceuticals was one of the first large proponents of extracting CBD and using it in medical trials.

GW was founded in 1998 and began their first clinical trials just one year later. Geoffrey Guy, a co-founder of GW, sought CBD-rich cannabis plants for isolation and cultivation. His belief was that by using CBD-rich plants, his company could produce a medicine made of cannabis that had little or no psychoactive effect. According to its website, GW works with cannabinoid scientists worldwide to "explore the potential of a range of novel cannabinoid molecules in a number of distinct therapeutic areas including epilepsy, glaucoma, and schizophrenia." GW's research has spurned more interest in the subject of medical marijuana and CBD, especially in the United States.

In 2003, the United States Department of Health was granted Patent No. 6,630,507 for "cannabiniods as antioxidants and neuroprotectants". A patent is a property right given to an inventor by the government. It allows the inventor "to exclude others from making, using, offering for sale, or selling the invention throughout the United States or importing the invention into the United States" for a limited amount of time. The summary of the patent filing for cannabinoids states that CBD and other cannabinoids have "surprisingly" been found to protect nerve cells from damage and to prevent oxidative stress, an imbalance between harmful free radicals and the body's ability to neutralize their effects.

According to the patent filing, the "object of this invention [is] to provide a new class of antioxidant drugs . . . by administering a therapeutically effective amount of a cannabinoid to a subject who has a disease caused by oxidative stress." This means that, should the use of cannabinoids become legal, the right to make and sell drugs made from cannabinoids is held by the Department of Health. The United States government is aware of the medical benefits of cannabis and the profits that can be made from such drugs, yet it has not removed cannabis from the list of Schedule I drugs from the Controlled Substances Act (CSA). This is yet another example of the government's own contradictory actions when it comes to cannabis and CBD. Unlike THC, CBD itself is not nor has it ever been listed formally in the CSA, a point not to be ignored.

Even though the government has not yet repealed the nationwide marijuana ban, it is looking into testing specific pharmaceutical drugs. One of GW's products, Epidiolex, was approved for use in clinical trials by the Food and Drug Administration (FDA) in 2015. This is important because, depending on the results of the trials, Epidiolex could become the first CBD-based prescription drug to be approved by the FDA. Epidiolex contains 98 percent of CBD as its active ingredient, with a purpose of treating children with a rare form of epilepsy called Lennox-Gastaut Syndrome.

In 2016, the results of Phase 3 of the clinical trials were released. In Phase

3, the drug was given to large groups of people, and various types of information about the drug, such as side effects, effectiveness, and comparisons to other treatments, were observed. The trial was randomized, double-blind, and placebo-controlled. The results found that patients taking Epidiolex experienced 37 percent less seizures per month, compared with patients taking a placebo, who experienced 17 percent less seizures per month.

In 2017, *The New England Journal of Medicine* published additional results on Epidiolex (98 percent plant-concentrated CBD). This trial showed that CBD reduced the frequency of convulsive seizures among children and young adults with Dravet syndrome over a 14-week period, but was associated with adverse events, including somnolence and elevation of liver-enzyme levels. Additional data is needed to determine the long-term efficacy and safety of CBD for Dravet Syndrome. Although Epidiolex is not a synthetic drug, it is missing most of the natural co-factors found in the original hemp medications, preparations, and ancient remedies made from the whole hemp plant.

Questions have also arisen about the multiple drug-to-drug interactions reported in this trial between CBD and the other anti-epileptic medications. Those drug interactions clearly illustrate that when isolating CBD to 98 percent and omitting the naturally occurring co-factors, as is required for the FDA drug approval process, that it is much less effective than agricultural hemp CBD oil products with 2 to 5 percent naturally-occurring CBD. That's because they're completely different products in two totally different markets with different customers. Epidiolex appears to be a breakthrough pharmaceutical drug, while agricultural hemp extracts, that are a source of natural CBD appear to be the most revolutionary dietary supplement to date.

Supplemental CBD

As a supplemental product, hemp CBD extracts are typically found in an oil form and are commonly sold in local independent health food stores, online, or in dispensaries. One of the first significant cases proving the effectiveness of CBD oil was that of Charlotte Figi. Her story was broadcast on the CNN news channel in 2013, drawing worldwide attention to the medical benefits of CBD products. Charlotte was five years old and suffering from over 300 grand mal seizures a week when her parents decided to give her CBD oil. They had previously tried pharmaceutical drugs and other medical procedures that did not provide significant help, and turned to CBD oil after watching a documentary about medical marijuana. Almost 100 percent of Charlotte's seizures were treated by the CBD oil.

A high-CBD, low-THC product named Charlotte's Web was named after

Charlotte Figi. It was developed in 2011 by six brothers who cross-bred a strain of marijuana with industrial hemp, resulting in a higher CBD level than most marijuana plants. They used these plants to extract their oil.

The government-run agency National Institutes of Health has acknowledged that CBD can have many benefits in treating a wide range of inflammatory-driven conditions, including depression, anxiety, obesity, and even cancer. Its information summary on cannabis and cannabinoids for use with cancer has covered the topics of cannabis as a relief for pain, nausea, anxiety, and as a way to curb the unpleasant side effects of chemotherapy, citing the results of several clinical studies. Even with this acknowledgment and without the force of law, the Drug Enforcement Agency (DEA) is suggesting that hemp CBD extracts are the same as a "marijuana extract" that falls under a Schedule I classification: "All extracts that contain CBD will also contain at least small amounts of other cannabinoids…such marijuana extracts remain in Schedule I." Although the exact wording of CBD is not and has never been listed as a Schedule I, the DEA's position on hemp CBD extracts appears to be defaulting again to its zero tolerance policy for THC, including the trace amount that naturally occurs in hemp.

Only Congress has the power to make law, not the DEA. Hemp products are already federally legal; however, questions surrounding the intellectual property and ultimately the fate of cannabis products, especially CBD, are to be determined by the courts.

Today, legally selling and purchasing CBD oil is a gray area: In some states that allow medical and recreational marijuana, these products are permitted. But on the federal level, things are a little different when discussing isolated CBD, which is awaiting formal FDA approval. As you learned on page 10, the only hemp and cannabis products free of all risk in the U.S. are those that contain absolutely no THC, not even the trace amounts already excluded from the CSA definition of marijuana and found in legal hemp products. That baffling contradiction is at the heart of the debate.

Nevertheless, the DEA still considers CBD oil a marijuana extract with no accepted medical use. Contrary to the DEA, the Food and Drug Administration considers CBD a "new drug" that must be used under doctor supervision and cannot be labeled a dietary supplement. Despite the uncertainty surrounding the legality of CBD, there is no question that CBD is beneficial in treating and managing many conditions.

CONCLUSION

It is unfortunate that after a long and proven track record, scare tactics and propaganda caused the downfall of hemp and cannabis. Hemp was once vital in the production of supplies and clothing in the U.S., while cannabis's medical benefits were touted. But by the 1930s, competing industries and politicians sought to destroy hemp and cannabis before placing a tax on and ultimately outlawing them. Market forces lead to the development of patentable medicines that inevitably replaced natural hemp extracts with the FDA approved synthetic cannabis drugs Dronabinol (Marinol) and Nabilone (Cesamet).

Today, however, natural hemp CBD extracts are gaining more interest and attention. While the research on CBD is still early, the information is promising. As CBD medications enter clinical testing and gain more attention, the stigma surrounding it may finally be forgotten. CBD can serve to benefit a new generation of patients; it has already been shown to kill cancer cells, relieve pain and nausea, curb anxiety, stop seizures, and so much more. In Chapter 2, you will learn more about the science behind this healing process.

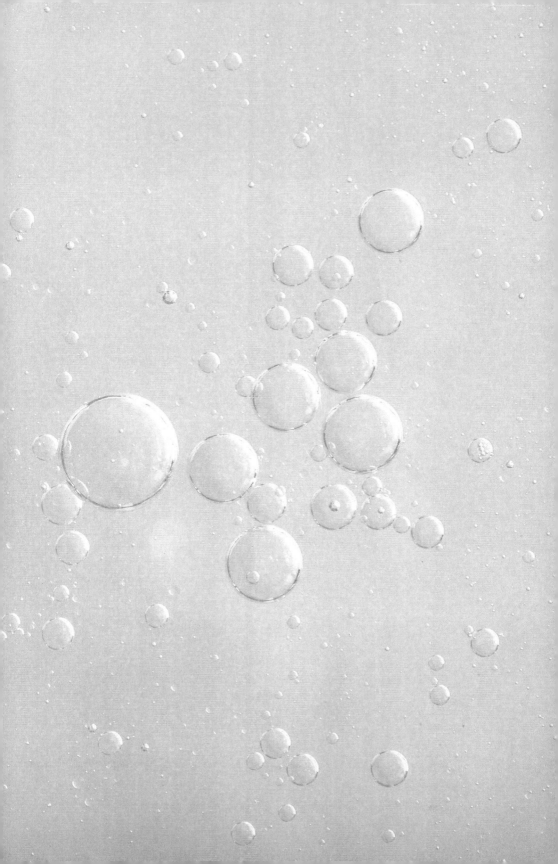

2.

The Science of CBD

In Chapter 1, you learned about the hemp plant's many uses throughout history. Hemp was an important part of societies all over the world; it was used for manufacturing, for food, and for healing. But political agendas have caused hemp's benefits to be ignored in favor of painting another plant in the family, marijuana, in a bad light. The proven medical benefits of hemp seemed to have been forgotten by the public. In this chapter, you will find out more about the science when it comes to hemp and CBD, and how they may help manage conditions such as epilepsy, depression, cancer, and much more.

HEMP BASICS

It is important to understand how the hemp plant works, how CBD is processed from it, and how hemp differs from marijuana. Both are variants of the cannabis plant, each cultivated with its own unique set of uses: Marijuana is grown specifically for its psychoactive and intoxicating properties, while hemp has been historically grown for its seed and fiber. This variance is due to slight differences in chemical makeup and DNA: both plants produce the cannabinoids THC and CBD in their buds and leaves, but while marijuana plants typically have a THC content of anywhere between 5 and 25 percent, true agricultural hemp has a negligible amount—usually less than 0.3% THC.

There are also some differences in appearance. Hemp grows to be much taller than marijuana. Hemp plants range from 10 to 15 feet in height, in contrast to about 5 feet for an average marijuana plant. Another difference is that marijuana plants grow "out" instead of "up." They tend to be bushier and fuller than hemp plants and need to be widely spaced apart so that the sunlight can more easily reach the buds. The tops and buds of both plants are similar in appearance, but marijuana buds tend have a bit of a "hairier" look to them.

Hemp plants range in size and reflect environmental conditions. Some have thin stalks, while other varieties are very thick with little vegetation, other than the flowering tops. When cultivators plant hemp, the amount of space they put between the hemp plants depends on whether the hemp is being grown for the fiber or the seed. When grown for the fiber, hemp plants are usually planted very close together; when grown for the seed, the plants can be spaced farther apart so that the seed-buds have more room to blossom.

In a 2013 conference with Congress, the DEA alleged that legalizing industrial hemp cultivation "would provide easy cover to hide more potent marijuana plants." This is simply not true. It would not be prudent to plant hemp and marijuana plants close together, because cross-pollination would render the plants infertile. A person trying to hide marijuana plants in a hemp field would end up with marijuana that has low THC and very weak psychoactive and intoxication effects. The marijuana would actually be *less* potent. This is why it is so important for policymakers to learn the differences between the two plants; legalizing hemp cultivation nationwide would not lead to more people getting high.

INDUSTRIAL HEMP IN THE UNITED STATES

In Chapter 1, you learned that the 2014 United States Farm Bill legalized the cultivation of industrial hemp in a certain number of states. Section 7606 of the Bill defines "industrial hemp" as a derivative of the cannabis sativa plant with a THC level that does not exceed 0.3 percent on a dry weight basis. The Bill permits industrial hemp to be grown, cultivated, and marketed for research and educational purposes. Below, we will discuss what kinds of materials are made from hemp and from what part of the plant they are produced.

The hemp plant is composed of several different parts, including the stalk (stem), the leaves, the roots, and the seeds. The hemp stalk perhaps has the widest range of uses. It can be processed to make textiles; for example, you have probably come across clothing or shoes made of hemp. Such clothing is considered more environmentally friendly than clothing made of cotton, because hemp is naturally pest-resistant. This eliminates the need for toxic chemical pesticides. The stalk can also transform into industrial or building materials, such as rope, caulking, fiberglass, insulation, or canvas. (The word *canvas* is actually derived from the word *cannabis*.) The herd inside the hemp stalk can be used to make paper.

Hemp seeds are often used in food, supplements, and cosmetics. They are hefty in the essential fatty acids omega-3 ALA and omega-6 LA that our bodies require but cannot make on their own. The seeds are used to make the popular hemp seed oil, a noted dietary supplement. Hemp seed oil is often called just "hemp oil." Note that this is *not* the same as hemp CBD oil or hemp extracts whose health benefits we discuss in this book. Hemp seed, however, does have valuable health effects of its own. (See "Hemp Seeds and Health" inset on page 19.)

Many people like to use hemp seed oil on their skin or in their hair because of its moisturizing properties. Hemp seed oil has also been used throughout history as a biofuel. The fuel it creates is free of pollutants and has four times the energy as corn-based ethanol. Some car manufacturers are working on ways to infuse hemp seed oil into their vehicle manufacturing to make cars more "green" and recyclable. Hemp-based protein powder can even be made from the seeds as a vegan-friendly alternative to animal proteins.

The leaves and flowers of the hemp plant are where the CBD component can be primarily found. Some CBD is also found in the stems, stalks, and raw seed oil. CO_2 extraction represents an environmentally friendly way to produce full spectrum, CBD-rich hemp extracts. The leaves are known for their absorbent nature and can be used as animal bedding or as compost and mulch. The roots can also be used for compost because of the nutrients they carry.

There are many strong arguments to support hemp legalization in all states. It's important to stress that hemp is *not* a drug and its products will not get anyone high. It is an important manufacturing and industrial

---

Hemp Seeds and Health

While CBD's legality has been met with uncertainty, a fully legal component of hemp that has its own benefits is the hemp seed. Hemp seeds that have been sterilized have no THC. They can be eaten raw, ground into meal, liquidized into milk or juice, or pressed into oil.

A 2017 study reported the potential anti-inflammatory effects of a substance found inside the hemp seed called grossamide. The researchers demonstrated that grossamide obstructed pro-inflammatory compounds in the body and concluded with a suggestion "that grossamide could be a potential therapeutic candidate for inhibiting neuroinflammation in neurodegenerative diseases."

In addition to the new research into grossamide, hemp seed has the tried-and-true benefit of providing you with the essential fatty acids (EFAs) that your body needs but cannot produce on its own. The most significant of these fatty acids are omega-3 and omega-6. By consuming optimal amounts of these substances, you can relieve joint pain, lower your triglyceride levels, enrich your brain cells, and offer dozens of other health benefits. Hemp seed oil is made of over 80 percent essential fatty acids!

substance, and an environment-friendly plant material that can be used in thousands of products. Hemp extracts that contain naturally-occurring CBD can be used in the relief of many health conditions, as you will learn below.

HOW CBD WORKS IN THE BODY

When you consume a hemp product made with CBD, you may wonder what the CBD does inside your body that allows it to exert its benefits. Cannabinoids like CBD interact with the body's *endocannabinoid system and other targets*. The endocannabinoid system, or ECS, is a network of cell receptors, molecules, and enzymes found in the brain and nervous systems that work together to perform specific functions. The ECS plays a role in a variety of psychological processes, including appetite, pain-sensation, anxiety, mood and memory.

Our bodies naturally make substances that participate in the ECS, called *endocannabinoids*. CBD, however, is not an endocannabinoid. Instead, it is a *phytocannabinoid:* a cannabinoid that comes from a plant. In the following sections, we will explain different parts of the ECS and how CBD affects each one.

Cell Receptors

A cell receptor is a protein molecule that is attached to the cell membrane. The receptor reacts to incoming chemical signals. Signal and receptor combinations can then determine the cell's activity. In the endocannabinoid system (ECS), the two main cannabinoid receptors are called CB1 and CB2. CB1 receptors are mostly found in the brain, nervous system, and certain organs and tissues, while CB2 is found mostly in white blood cells. New research has also discovered CB2 receptors in certain brain regions. CBD does not directly bind often with these receptors, but it does exert some interesting effects on them. CBD also interacts with other receptors, as you will learn in the following sections.

CB1 and CB2 Receptors

The highest levels of the CB1 receptor are found in the brain, particularly in the hippocampus, cerebral cortex, cerebellum, and the basal ganglia. These parts of the brain are in charge of your motor movements and behaviors, cognition, short-term memory, attention span, language, balance, and much more. This means that these functions are most affected by cannabis intake. THC—the psychoactive component in marijuana—binds directly to CB1 but CBD does not. Instead, CBD works to *prevent* THC's bond with CB1.

Take the example of a person who ingests a high-CBD, low-THC product. He will not feel high because, not only is the THC level low, but the CBD is interacting with the CB1 receptors in his body. The CBD is sending a chemical message to the receptor, directing the receptor to change shape. When the receptor's shape changes, its ability to make a perfect bond with THC declines. THC's psychoactive effects will not be strong, if they even appear at all.

Meanwhile, the CB2 receptor is located primarily in the white blood cells. White blood cells are the director of your immune system because they protect you from infections and foreign manner. While studies have shown that THC has an effect on the CB2 receptor, much less is known about CBD's effect on CB2. It is believed that CBD indirectly communicates with CB2.

Other Receptors

CB1 and CB2 may be the main receptors in the endocannabinoid system, but several other receptors play important roles in the body. CBD reacts with receptors called 5-HT1A, TRPV1, GPR55, and GABA-A. These names may sound mechanical, but we will break them down into simple terms and explain how each affects your health. We will also describe how CBD interacts with each receptor. These are far from the only receptors that interact with CBD, but they are some of the most notable.

5-HT1A Receptor

The 5-HT1A receptor can be found in most of the same parts of the brain as the CB1 receptor. Some of the functions it affects are your mood, appetite, sleep patterns, and pain perception. It is part of a family of receptors that are sometimes called "serotonin receptors," named after the neurotransmitter that boosts feelings of happiness. Serotonin activates these receptors. However, CBD can also directly activate the 5-HT1A receptor. A study on animals in 2014 demonstrated that CBD's interaction with 5-HT1A caused anti-depressant and anti-anxiety effects.

TRPV-1 Receptor

TRPV-1 is mostly present in the peripheral nervous system, which connects the central nervous system in the brain with the rest of the body. Specifically, TRPV-1 is involved with relaying and mediating pain, inflammation, and your body temperature. CBD binds to and stimulates TRPV-1, leading to pain relief. To further explain, CBD is believed to actually desensitize the TRPV-1 receptor. This action can be helpful in treating conditions where TRPV-1 sensitivity is heightened, such as rheumatoid arthritis. The study that reported these findings concluded "the nontoxic and nonpsychoactive compound CBD may represent a useful pharmacological alternative in the treatment of the disease-associated chronic pain."

GPR55 Receptor

The GPR55 receptor is expressed in the cerebellum part of the brain and in bone-building cells called osteoblasts. It is sometimes called the "orphan receptor" because researchers do not know if it is a part of a broader family of receptors. GPR55 helps to balance blood pressure and bone density. When this receptor is disrupted, it can overreact, leading to conditions such as osteoporosis, cancer, and obesity. Ruth Ross, a scientist at the University of Aberdeen, has noted that CBD is an antagonist of GPR55. This means that CBD can stop GPR55 from over-signaling.

GABA-A Receptor

Similar to the way CBD changes the shape of the CB1 receptor, CBD can also change the shape of the GABA-A receptor. GABA-A normally binds with GABA, which is short for gamma-Aminobutyric acid. GABA is a neurotransmitter that has a calming effect on the body. When CBD changes the shape of the GABA-A receptor, this calming effect is strengthened. A study published in 2017 tested the effect of CBD on GABA receptors to find out if their relationship could explain CBD's anti-epileptic, anti-anxiety, and pain relieving features. The authors concluded that their "...results reveal a mode of action of CBD on specifically configured GABA-A receptors that may be relevant to the anticonvulusant [anti-seizure] and anxiolytic [anti-anxiety] effects of the compound."

CBD SAFETY

Many people are hesitant to consume or support the use of CBD because of the conflicting information regarding its safety. However, a number of studies have found CBD to be generally well tolerated and safe for consumption, even in high doses and with chronic use. A 2011 review of over 130 studies and papers about CBD summarized:

> CBD is non-toxic in non-transformed cells and does not induce changes on food intake, does not induce catalepsy, does not affect . . . heart rate, blood pressure and body temperature, does not affect gastrointestinal transit and does not alter psychomotor or psychological functions. Also, chronic use and high doses up to 1,500 mg/day of CBD are reportedly well tolerated in humans.

This review looked at studies that tested CBD's effects on both animals and humans. The studies were a mix of *in vivo* tests conducted on living creatures and *in vitro* tests performed on cells outside of their normal biological environment.

In these studies, CBD was not found to have any significant side effects, even with a wide range of doses. It did not interfere with important psychomotor and psychological functions; subjects who participated in a verbal paired-associate learning test did not have their results affected by the use of CBD. Studies of more chronic use of CBD found that it was well-tolerated across several healthy and ill populations. It did not affect patients' neurological, clinical, psychiatric, blood, or urine examinations. Several patients with psychiatric disorders, including schizophrenia and bipolar disorder, displayed extremely positive results after using CBD daily for three to four weeks. Their psychotic symptoms were reduced and they experienced fewer side effects than what they had experienced under prescription drugs.

CBD was also tested on patients with Parkinson's disease in a four-week clinical trial. The CBD doses ranged from 150 mg to 400 mg a day and were given in conjunction with the patients' usual treatments. At the end of the four weeks, the study found that there were no serious side effects, cognitive and motor symptoms experienced no change, and the patients' psychotic symptoms were notably reduced. Taking this information in combination with the results from the study of schizophrenic patients, it seems CBD has the potential to strongly reduce psychotic symptoms.

Interactions

Although CBD has not been shown to directly interact with pharmaceutical drugs, some concern lies in the way CBD interacts with certain liver enzymes. This family of liver enzymes, called cytochrome P450 or CYP, metabolizes most pharmaceutical drugs. It is thought that more than 60 percent of drugs on the market are broken down by CYP.

Certain doses of CBD deactivate these enzymes, although the exact dose has not been determined. CBD competes with the CYP enzymes for the same sites in the liver. The two components displace and deactivate each other. CYP is then unable to metabolize other substances.

However, the degree to which CBD interacts with CYP enzymes varies widely depending on a number of factors. The amount of CBD consumed, the form (pill/capsule, paste, balm, etc) in which it is consumed, the strength of the CBD, the genetic makeup of the person consuming the CBD, and more can affect how CBD competes with the CYP enzymes. Different pharmaceutical drugs seem to be affected in different ways, as well: In one clinical trial, a

25 mg oral dose of pure isolated CBD was found to influence the metabolism of an anti-seizure drug. On the contrary, CBD induces CYP1A1, which is responsible for degradation of cancerogenic substances such as benzopyrene. CYP1A1 can be found in the intestine and CBD- induced higher activity could therefore prevent absorption of cancerogenic substances into the bloodstream and thereby help to protect DNA. Another clinical trial found that a 40 mg sublingual dose of a CBD-rich spray had no effect on the CYP enzymes.

More research needs to be conducted in this area before making a clear determination as to exactly how well CBD interacts with pharmaceutical drugs. For now, it seems safest to avoid mixing more than 15 mg of CBD per day with multiple pharmaceutical medications, without the consent of your physician.

Enhancing CBD's Effects

Taken by itself, isolated CBD is not absorbed very effectively by the body. Researchers and enthusiasts are looking into substances that can be combined with CBD to enhance its bioavailability (the dosage level that reaches the circulation and has an active effect on the body). Evidence is suggesting that oral co-administration of lipids enhances the systemic exposure of rats to THC and CBD by 2.5 fold and 3 fold, respectively compared to lipid free formulas. Look for CBD products with lipid carriers like extra virgin olive oil).

CONCLUSION

In this chapter, you learned about the science behind hemp and CBD. Hemp and marijuana have distinctive qualities and perform different functions. Hemp is an extremely useful plant for many reasons, and researchers should be allowed to cultivate it and study its healing benefits without fear of repercussion. So far, we at least know about some of the receptors in our bodies with which CBD extract from hemp interacts. These CBD-receptor interactions can help relieve symptoms of depression, anxiety, pain, inflammation, osteoporosis, and more. In Part II, we will explore specific conditions and explain the benefits CBD has on each one.

3.

Legal Status
of Hemp and CBD Oil

n previous chapters, we touched upon the legal status of hemp, CBD, and the remedies that are made from these substances. The current laws covering cannabis—which control the growth and distribution of both marijuana and hemp—have been evolving over the past several decades. But while for most of the twentieth century, the political and legal movement was all in the direction of restrictions and prohibitions, since the onset of the new millennium, there has been rapid movement towards legalization.

In this chapter, we will examine the history of cannabis laws and explain how it has led us to modern laws. We will take a closer look at the various contradictions and unclear statements in the law and review some of the major studies that analyze the effects of legal medical marijuana. With every passing year, more lenient medical marijuana laws pass in different states; despite the controversy-laden past, the future looks to be bright for hemp, CBD, medical marijuana, and for all of the patients who can benefit.

FORMING THE FEDERAL BUREAU OF NARCOTICS

The view of cannabis as a dangerous substance began to gain traction once the government started its fight against opiates and narcotics in the early twentieth century. At this point in time, opiates and narcotics—such as cocaine, heroin, and morphine—were more popular than cannabis (see "Drug Addiction in the Twentieth Century" inset on page 29). Lawmakers were attempting to regulate and limit distribution and sale of drugs and alcohol, with varying degrees of success.

In 1914, Congress passed the Harrison Narcotics Tax Act. This was the first Federal law to regulate the medical use and criminalize the non-medical use of drugs, essentially setting the stage for stricter laws in the years to come. The Harrison Act imposed taxes and regulations on the manufacture and distribution of opiates. Physicians, naturopaths, pharmacists, and other healers had to pay a tax and become licensed to prescribe and sell such drugs. It was unlawful for anyone to possess these drugs unless they had paid the tax and obtained the license or the drugs had been prescribed to them by a wide variety of licensed physicians.

Although the Harrison Act outlined the penalties for violation of the law, it did not give states the power to actually seize illegal drugs. The law was more focused on penalizing people for tax evasion—indeed, its official title was "An Act to provide for the registration of, with collectors of internal revenue, and to impose a special tax upon all persons who [deal in] opium or coca leaves."

As officials cracked down on opiate, narcotic, and cocaine use—as well as alcohol use—smoking cannabis started to gain popularity as a recreational activity. During and after the Mexican Revolution (1910–1920), the United States experienced a surge in immigrants from Mexico. With new migrants came age-old traditions; a new Spanish word, "marihuana," entered our vocabulary. "Marihuana," of course, is just another word for the cannabis plants that had been used for millennia. However, politicians and officials with a nationalist agenda seized on this unfamiliar word to start a propaganda campaign against Mexican immigrants.

Many newspapers labeled these immigrants as violent, disruptive, dangerous, and lazy. The "marihuana" some of them used recreationally was accused of being the source of this deviant behavior. Powerful businessmen like William Randolph Hearst took whatever opportunities they could to publish cartoons and articles berating cannabis and Mexicans.

The Federal Bureau of Narcotics was established in 1930 to enforce the Harrison Act. However, the FBN found the old law unsuitable for its purposes and pushed to have it replaced. In 1934, the FBN passed the Uniform State Narcotic Drug Act. This new Act met demand for a nationwide, uniform law to prosecute those who held narcotics (e.g., heroin, morphine, and opium) illegally. While it still focused on narcotics, a conditional proposition for cannabis was added: "Any state wishing to regulate sale and possession of marijuana was instructed to simply add cannabis to the definition of 'narcotic drugs.'" This allowed cannabis to be treated in the same matter as narcotics if the state so wished. This marked the beginning of cannabis regulation.

HARRY ANSLINGER AND PROPOGANDA

The FBN's first leader was Harry Anslinger, who was perhaps the most outspoken activist of cannabis prohibition, although the reasons why he so vehemently opposed cannabis are not clear. Prior to his role at the FBN, Anslinger had been the captain of the railroad police for the Pennsylvania

Drug Addiction in the Early Twentieth Century

While most of us are familiar with the anti-alcohol movement—which led to the Eighteenth Amendment of 1919, prohibiting the production and sale of alcohol—few are aware of the drug problems that co-existed in the early 1900s. Numerous concoctions containing cocaine, heroin, and morphine had been commonly used by healers for centuries to relieve pain and many other health disorders throughout the world. In Western cultures, medical doctors, osteopaths, naturopaths, druggists, dentists, herbalists, or anyone who claimed to be a healer could offer potions laced with these opiates. And not only were these products—such as laudanum (a tincture of opium)—commonly found on pharmacy shelves, "snake oil" salesmen travelled the countryside selling the same addictive products—guaranteeing "cures" and repeat customers.

By the late 1800s, smoking opium was becoming popular as a means to relax. Just as bars in Western cultures had become places to drink alcohol and socialize, the Chinese had established opium dens in many major cities in Europe, North America, and Australia. Initially catering to Chinese workers, these storefront dens began to quickly attract non-Chinese patrons. In England, Canada, and the United States, the use of opium was growing. The use of any of these hard drugs in medications or as a relaxant was legal. By 1900, a number of local ordinances were passed in cities such as San Francisco and New York City, but few were enforced.

At this time, as the anti-alcohol movement began to grow, drinking was promoted as an immoral behavior leading to the destruction of families, prostitution, and a number of other vices. Opiate use was viewed in a similar way, but with a major difference: it was seen more as a "Chinese problem"—that is, an ethnic problem. As time went on, this action of singling out an ethnic group as the source responsible for drug sales greatly influenced government drug policies on all levels.

Initially, the Harrison Narcotics Tax Act of 1914 was designed to control the sale of opiates and coca leaves to the various healing professions and druggists through their required registration with the government. However, as the FBN's powers were expanded to include any "narcotic drugs," they could now seize whatever they saw as an "illegal drug." Now, in the early twenty-first century, the same attitude seems to persist in many federal agencies in spite of the research and science regarding hemp.

Railroad and the assistant commissioner for the Treasury Department's Bureau of Prohibition. He was known as an honest figure who sought to bring down corruption. Some critics say he wanted to maintain this reputation after the failure of alcohol Prohibition in the 1920s. Another theory is that he was acting in support of industries that competed with hemp, such as synthetic fibers and timber. Evidence exists that he may have been motivated by racism, as well.

Regardless of his reasons, Anslinger was successful in turning the country against cannabis. Interestingly, before the alcohol Prohibition was lifted, he stated that cannabis was harmless and not a problem. But after Prohibition ended, he began to ignore many doctors' and researchers' reports that marijuana had no connection to crime rates. He exaggerated the effect marijuana had on a person's sanity, claiming it was "a short cut to the insane asylum." His compilation of 200 crimes, called the "Gore Files," blamed cannabis use for each and every one of the crimes. However, researchers later proved cannabis was *not* the cause of 198 of these 200 crimes. The remaining two stories couldn't be disproved only because no records of those crimes existed.

The 1936 propaganda film *Reefer Madness* further pushed the message that marijuana would cause young people to commit murder and suicide, hallucinate, "live in sin," and become addicted to the drug. African-American jazz musicians also became scapegoats. Government officials, led by Anslinger, started a vendetta against black musicians. They claimed that cannabis caused "men of color to become violent and solicit sex from white women." Anslinger even had the famed jazz singer Billie Holiday arrested on her deathbed—where she was clearly not a danger to anybody else—for cannabis possession.

With Americans now sufficiently fearful of cannabis, the stage was set to pass a new federal law to impede its spread. In 1928, the International Opium Convention had ruled cannabis a "drug" instead of a prescribed "medicine." Notably, the Convention called cannabis by the name "Indian hemp." Anslinger used this decision, along with other hearings on the subject, to propose a new and more restrictive bill almost ten years later—the Marijuana Tax Act, lumping marijuana and hemp together.

THE MARIJUANA TAX ACT

The Marijuana Tax Act was passed in 1937. Under this law, anyone who handled cannabis—in other words, anyone who sold, dealt, prescribed, gave away, or dispensed marijuana or hemp—had to register with the FBN and purchase a one-dollar tax stamp. If a handler failed to do this, he faced up to a $2,000 fine and/or prison time. Although the 1932 Uniform State Narcotic Drug Act allowed states to regulate cannabis if they chose, the Marijuana Tax Act, for all intents and purposes, criminalized cannabis across the nation.

The Marijuana Tax Act also provided an outline as to exactly which parts of the plant were to be regulated. It determined that "marihuana" included the seeds, the resin, and "every compound, manufacture, salt, derivative, mixture, or preparation of such plant, its seeds or resin." It excluded the plant's stalks, fiber from stalks, oil from sterilized seeds, or any product made of stalks or fiber.

Despite the support for the Marijuana Tax Act, there were also many detractors. As we mentioned in Chapter 1, the American Medical Association stated it had no reason to believe cannabis was dangerous. Fiorello La Guardia, then the mayor of New York, was also opposed to the Act. He enlisted the New York Academy of Medicine to publish a report detailing the effects of smoking marijuana. After five years of research, the "LaGuardia Committee" found in their study that—contrary to what the Federal government claimed—"juvenile delinquency is not associated with the practice of smoking marijuana…the publicity concerning the catastrophic effects of marijuana smoking…is unfounded." Harry Anslinger dismissed the report as "unscientific," despite the number of doctors and researchers that had worked on the report.

HEMP AND WORLD WAR II

Even as a domestic war against marijuana raged on, industrial hemp enjoyed resurgence during World War II (1939–1945). There was a shortage in imported industrial fibers normally used to be used in the manufacturing of rope, cords, parachutes, and other materials. Because of this, farmers were encouraged to grow hemp in support of the American soldiers fighting in the war. The farmers were given incentives for growing the hemp, such as exemption from the war draft.

A fourteen-minute promotional film called *Hemp for Victory* was released in 1942 by the United States Department of Agriculture (USDA). The film described hemp's use throughout history as an industrial material. It also explained the best methods for growing and harvesting hemp. The goal was to have 50,000 acres of hemp plants by 1943.

Of course, since hemp and cannabis were still being taxed under the Marijuana Tax Act, the film warned farmers: "This is hemp seed. Be careful how you use it. For you to grow hemp legally, you must have a federal registration and tax stamp. This is provided for in your contract. Ask your county agent about it. Don't forget."

The "Hemp for Victory" campaign was short-lived; by 1945, the war had ended and many farmers were faced with cancelled contracts and acres of hemp that were no longer needed. By 1958, hemp cultivation had essentially ceased.

OVERTURNING THE MARIJUANA TAX ACT

The Marijuana Tax Act was in place for about thirty years and made it financially difficult to grow hemp. This tax effectively eliminated legal cannabis and hemp cultivation. Cannabis and marijuana were taboo substances and many citizens believed they were harmful. However, the legality of the law was finally decided by the Supreme Court in 1969, during the case *Leary v. United States*.

Dr. Timothy Leary was a professor at Harvard University. On December 22, 1965, he attempted to drive into Mexico from Texas with his two teenage children and his girlfriend for a vacation. Their car was denied entry at the Mexican customs station and they drove back into Texas. There, the American customs inspector asked to search the car and found what appeared to be traces of marijuana on the car floor and glove compartment. Upon further scrutiny, the inspector found a small box containing marijuana cigarettes in Leary's daughter's clothing. Leary took responsibility for the drugs and was arrested in violation of the Marijuana Tax Act. He was sentenced to thirty years in prison, a $30,000 fine, and an order to seek psychiatric treatment.

Leary appealed this sentence on the basis that the Marijuana Tax Act was unconstitutional because it violated his Fifth Amendment rights. The Fifth Amendment protects citizens from self-incrimination. The Marijuana Tax Act required "all transfers of marijuana" to be recorded with an order form. Leary argued that if he had abided and requested an order form, he would have identified himself as part of "a selective group inherently suspect of criminal activities." The Supreme Court ultimately agreed and the Act was overturned. However, it would only be a year until it was replaced by another law prohibiting cannabis.

In 1968, a year before the Supreme Court decision was handed down, the FBN was merged with Bureau of Drug Abuse Control, an agency of the Food and Drug Administration, to form the Bureau of Narcotics and Dangerous Drugs (BNDD). The BNDD was later merged into what is now the Drug Enforcement Administration (DEA) in 1973.

THE CONTROLLED SUBSTANCES ACT

In 1970, the Comprehensive Drug Abuse Prevention and Control Act was signed by President Richard Nixon. Its basic purpose was to restrict the availability of certain drugs by requiring the drugs to be tightly secured and monitored by pharmacies. Title II of this Act was called the Controlled Substances Act (CSA). This is the part of the law that divided drugs into five schedules. (See inset "Drug Schedules" below.) Cannabis was categorized as a Schedule I drug—meaning that the government found it to be highly addictive and to have no proven medical use. Cannabis was now illegal to manufacture, distribute, or possess under the federal law. The only exception is if the cannabis is dispensed and/or possessed as part of a federally approved research program.

The CSA exempts certain parts of the cannabis plant—the stalk, fiber, and sterilized seeds—from the definition of "marijuana." These parts of the plant do not have a significant amount of THC but do contain CBD, and when CO_2 is extracted, provide the opening to import hemp CBD oil from Europe. This provision allows preparations made from these parts, such as fabric or hemp seed oil, to be legally produced. When the DEA was formed in 1973, it was given the responsibility of enforcing the new federal drug laws—as well as consolidating and coordinating the government's drug control activities. Still, to the newly formed DEA, the specifics of what was legal to grow and what was not was more a matter of opinion than law.

Despite over thirty states passing their own laws decriminalizing or legalizing marijuana, the plant remains illegal on the federal level as of 2017.

UNDERSTANDING THE "VAGUE" CRITERIA OF THE CSA

You may be wondering why cannabis and its extracts are determined to have "no currently accepted medical use," when there are countless studies and anecdotes that prove their benefits. As it turns out, this phrase is not officially defined in the Controlled Substances Act. The DEA later developed its own criteria for what it means for a substance to have "accepted medical use:"

- Its chemical makeup must be known and able to be reproduced.

- "Adequate safety studies" and "adequate and well-controlled studies proving efficacy" must exist.

- "Qualified experts" must accept it.

- "Scientific evidence" must be widely available.

As you can see, this criteria is not very specific nor is it written in the original law, but it has been upheld in court cases, such as *Alliance for Cannabis*

Therapeutics v. DEA in 1994. For a substance to receive "approved medical use" status, it must be approved by the FDA. Researchers face many obstacles in attempting to prove medical benefit, however. There is only one federal supplier of research marijuana, meaning that the only legal supply is spread thin across different research groups. The process to apply for this research marijuana is lengthy and involves contacting three to four different government agencies. Universities and laboratories may not have federal funding for cannabis research; some may be uncomfortable with conducting controversial research. As more and more states begin to legalize medical and recreational cannabis, the pressure is on for the Federal government to provide more resources to researchers.

Drug Schedules

The Controlled Substances Act of 1970 established five categories, or "schedules," of drugs. Drugs are categorized by how addictive they are, their abuse potential, and their proven medical benefits (if any). The legality of the drugs range from illegal to prescription-only to available over-the-counter. According to the DEA, the schedules are classified as follows:

Schedule I. Schedule I drugs have no currently accepted medical use, a high potential for abuse, and are illegal. Examples include heroin, LSD, marijuana (cannabis), and ecstasy.

Schedule II. Schedule II drugs have a high potential for abuse and dependency and are considered dangerous. Most are prescription-only and some are illegal. Examples include cocaine, methamphetamine, methadone, and medications such as Vicodin, OxyContin, Adderall, and Ritalin.

Schedule III. Schedule III drugs have a moderate to low potential for physical or psychological addiction. Examples include ketamine, steroids, testosterone, and medications containing less than 90 mg of codeine per dose.

Schedule IV. Schedule IV drugs have a low risk of dependence or abuse. Examples include the medications Xanax, Ambien, Valium, Ativan, and Darvocet.

Schedule V. Schedule V drugs have a lower potential for dependence or abuse than Schedule IV drugs and contain limited quantities of narcotics. Examples include most cough syrups and medications such as Lomotil, Motofen, and Lyrica.

MODERN LAWS

In the new millennium, cannabis has begun a slow redemption. Hemp is being cultivated in the U.S. again, with some limitations. Marijuana and/or CBD are permitted in over two dozen states. (See "State Medical Marijuana Laws" below.)

There now exists two sets of laws designed to control the growth and uses of cannabis and its extracts: the federal law, and the newly enacted state laws. Unfortunately, these laws are contradictory, making for a great deal of confusion. What this means is that it is possible to live in a state that has legalized marijuana, and still be prosecuted under the federal law. While there has not been strict enforcement of shipments in the United States, the United States and Canadian governments have seized packages of cannabinoid products in the past.

State Medical Marijuana Laws

Individual state laws range from legalization of both recreational and medical marijuana to decriminalized possession laws. "Decriminalized" means that while it is not legal, the penalties are lessened. Some states allow only medical marijuana to be sold or possessed with a doctor's permission, while some states have legalized recreational marijuana. Certain states only allow cannabis products that are low-THC and high-CBD for medical purposes.

California became the first state to allow medical marijuana in 1996. As of November 2016, eight states and Washington, D.C., have fully legal recreational and medical marijuana available for purchase and possession. Twelve states have legalized medical marijuana and decriminalized (but not legalized) the possession of recreational marijuana. Thirteen states have legal psychoactive medical cannabis, and another thirteen only have legal non-psychoactive (i.e., high-CBD) medical marijuana. Taken altogether, only three states—Idaho, South Dakota, and Kansas—prohibit cannabis completely. For more information about state laws, see the *Resources* on page 113.

Status of Hemp

The Marijuana Tax Act excluded industrial hemp from the definition of marijuana. However, when Congress repealed the Act in favor of the Controlled Substances Act, it abolished the distinction between hemp and marijuana, but it distinguished the non-psychoactive parts of the cannabis plant from the definition of marijuana. Currently, the federal definition of marijuana excludes the mature stalks of the plant; fiber produced from the stalks; oil or cake made from the seeds; any other compound, manufacture, salt, derivative, mixture, or preparation of such mature stalks (except the resin extracted therefrom), fiber, oil, or cake, or the sterilized seed of such plant, which is incapable of germination.

For decades, the United States has permitted importation of non-psychoactive hemp and hemp products exempted under the CSA. Importation of hemp and derivative products, including oil from hemp seeds, is consistent with decades-old business practices.

Federal jurisprudence legalizes non-psychoactive hemp products as exempt from the CSA. In *Hemp Industries Ass'n v. Drug Enforcement Administration*, the United States Court of Appeals for the Ninth Circuit invalidated regulations promulgated by the DEA that would have banned the manufacture and sale of edible products made from hemp seed and oil as substances controlled under the CSA. The Court affirmed that non-psychoactive hemp products do not contain any controlled substance as defined by the CSA. The Ninth Circuit's order enjoined DEA from engaging in enforcement actions against these products. Never overturned, the ruling remains good federal law and legal authority for distributing hemp-derived products. For this reason, distributors have continued to import non-psychoactive hemp from overseas, to trade in it, and to use it in the manufacture of products.

Despite legal permission for importation, until recently, Congress prohibited domestic growth and cultivation of industrial hemp. At the turn of the new millennium, however, domestic permissions emerged. Once thought of as an importer-only, the United States has since embraced local growth and cultivation of industrial hemp in its federal jurisprudence and statutory law.

On February 7, 2014, President Barack Obama signed the Farm Bill. Section 7606 – now common parlance in the hemp industry – provides for the "Legitimacy of Industrial Hemp Research." The Farm Bill, current federal law, is both limited in its reach and sweeping in its impact: It is limited to the extent that the use and production of industrial hemp is restricted to agricultural pilot programs conducted by state departments of agriculture, institutions of higher education, and/or their contractual designees. Therefore, the Farm Bill's provisions do not permit the growth or cultivation of industrial hemp outside the context of an agricultural pilot program, including on the tribal lands of American Indians.

It is sweeping to the extent that industrial hemp grown or cultivated within the context of an agricultural pilot program is exempt from other federal laws. In other words, federal laws that might otherwise restrict, regulate, or prohibit the use or production of industrial hemp, including the CSA, do not apply.

The Farm Bill also enumerates an important precedent: defining industrial hemp as "any part" of the cannabis plant. This standard legitimizes and legalizes all parts of the cannabis plant, including flowers, seeds, and stalks, so long as the product does not exceed three-tenths percent (0.3 percent) THC content.

The Farm Bill was not enacted without controversy. In the months following its enactment, federal agencies—most prominently the DEA—misinterpreted its meaning and application. The DEA initially raised objections to the importation of hemp seed for pilot programs. It took the position that such importation, as well as the cultivation of industrial hemp, would remain subject to the CSA and would require licenses (permits).

The Kentucky Department of Agriculture brought suit in federal district court to compel the DEA to release a shipment of hemp seed without a license. The litigation was settled informally in a manner that permitted seed importation and cultivation. In 2015, 125 pilot programs were authorized in Kentucky. Similar settlements have been reached between the DEA and departments of agriculture in other states that have legalized the growth and cultivation of industrial hemp.

Unfortunately, this ad hoc negotiation produced a patchwork of standards when it comes to federal regulation of industrial hemp. To eliminate confusion and provide clarity regarding the reach of the Farm Bill, Congress passed critical language in the Consolidated Appropriations Act for Fiscal Year 2016 ("Omnibus Law"). The Omnibus Law prohibits agencies, including the DEA, from expending federally-appropriated monies to interfere with or otherwise frustrate agricultural pilot programs established under the Farm Bill. The prohibition against interference extends to intrastate and interstate transportation, processing, sales, and use of industrial hemp grown or cultivated pursuant to the Farm Bill.

Taken together, the Ninth Circuit's order in *Hemp Industries Ass'n v. Drug Enforcement Administration* and the Farm Bill and Omnibus Law constitute an expansive, permissive federal legalization regime for industrial hemp. These authorities legitimize industrial hemp and derivative products and immobilize federal agencies that might otherwise pursue enforcement.

Most recently, the Industrial Hemp Farming Act of 2017 was introduced in Congress, with bipartisan support in both chambers. If passed, this Act would "amend the Controlled Substances Act to exclude industrial hemp from the definition of 'marijuana.'" Any cannabis plant with a THC level under 0.3 percent would be removed from the list of Schedule I drugs. As of 2017, this Act is still being reviewed in Congress and has not yet been deliberated.

DEA Ruling on Marijuana Extracts

With the state laws conflicting with federal law and the different allowances given to CBD extract, it is difficult to determine whether CBD is a legal substance. The term "CBD" is not included in the Controlled Substances Act, but is it included with marijuana and cannabis as a Schedule I drug? According to the Drug Enforcement Administration (DEA), the answer is yes.

In December 2016, the DEA announced a new code in the law. The name of this code is "Drug Code 7350—Establishment for a new code for marijuana extract." This amendment states that all cannabinoids would be considered illegal Schedule I drugs. There are over sixty cannabinoids in cannabis—CBD is one of them—and over 480 other natural compounds.

The announcement of this new code again raised concerns in the industrial hemp industry. While the manufacturers in this industry do not make products containing THC, many of their businesses rely on CBD-rich products. These manufacturers are allowed to operate on the provisions of the 2014 Farm Bill (see page 11), which exempted industrial hemp from the Controlled Substances Act. As a response to DEA, the Hemp Industries Association filed a federal lawsuit in January 2017.

HIA Lawsuit Against DEA

The Hemp Industries Association (HIA) is a nonprofit trade group that represents the businesses, farmers, and researchers who work with industrial hemp. In January 2017, the HIA filed a lawsuit against the DEA, accusing it of abusing its authority by not following the necessary procedures for scheduling new drugs under the Controlled Substances Act. Because the DEA did not follow the correct steps, the HIA says there is no legal basis for the new code and that the government cannot enforce it.

In its case, the HIA states what you already know by now: CBD has health benefits and is not psychoactive, nor is it intoxicating or habit forming. However, it is still looped in with THC because both substances come from the same plant. According to the HIA, CBD and other cannabinoids are not independently scheduled under federal law and so cannot be treated like Schedule I drugs. (The Schedule I law only includes THC and "marijuana," not "marijuana extracts.") The DEA, meanwhile, states that cannabinoids, including CBD, are subject to Schedule I classification because they are found in parts of the cannabis plant that are governed by the Controlled Substances Act.

POTENTIAL EFFECTS OF LEGALIZATION

Studies have been conducted in "legal" states to evaluate the effects of legalizing medical and/or recreational cannabis. The findings so far are very encouraging when you consider all of the propaganda that has been spread about cannabis in the past. Contrary to what has been said for decades, cannabis use does not increase the rate of violent crime. Researchers examined the FBI's violent crime data from 1990 to 2006 in eleven medical marijuana states. After analysis, they found that homicide and assault rates decreased by 2.4 percent for every year after medical marijuana became legal in these states. There was no increase in robbery or burglary. Their study concluded that medical marijuana laws were "not found to have a crime-enhancing effect" for the crimes studied: homicide, rape, robbery, assault, burglary, larceny, and automobile theft. A theory they gave to explain this was that people may substitute marijuana for alcohol, a substance that generally increases rates of crime.

To debunk another claim, opioid use and abuse do not rise in legal cannabis states. Several studies have found that cannabis is not a "gateway" to harder drugs. It may, in fact, curb opioid dependence since people can turn to medical marijuana instead of highly addictive opioids to manage pain and other medical conditions. States that have legal medical marijuana saw an average decrease of 23 percent in hospitalization rates for painkiller abuse and addiction, and an average 13 percent drop in hospitalization rates for opioid overdoses.

While drug-induced traffic fatalities have surpassed alcohol-related deaths, studies have shown a reduced number of such deaths in states where cannabis is legal. A study published in 2013 examined alcohol consumption and traffic fatality data from 1990 to 2010. The authors found that "MMLs (medical marijuana laws) are associated with decreases in the probability of [an individual] having consumed alcohol in the past month, binge drinking, and the number of drinks consumed." They also found that traffic fatalities fell 8 to 11 percent in the year after medical marijuana was legalized. They concluded that legalizing medical marijuana led to less people driving drunk (the leading cause of traffic fatalities), although the information does not necessarily mean that driving under the influence of marijuana is safer than driving under the influence of alcohol. A study looking at traffic fatalities from 1985–2014 discovered that such deaths dropped 11 percent in legal medical marijuana states.

The CBD component of cannabis plays a large role in these statistics. A review of twenty-one studies concluded that CBD interacts with receptors in the brain in a way that blocked the "reward-facilitating effect" that opioid use can bring to addicts. CBD also reduced some painful withdrawal symptoms. While more research needs to be conducted on CBD's specific role in medical marijuana laws' effects on society, the evidence so far is promising. CBD and medical cannabis, when used instead of alcohol and painkillers, can reduce violent crime and restrain the opioid addiction epidemic.

CONCLUSION

As more and more studies emerge that prove the benefits of medical marijuana and hemp extracts, and CBD, it is clear that the federal law needs to be updated. The government has the ability to, once and for all, remove the stigma of possessing a helpful but illegal healing substance. Because the DEA is conflicted about hemp CBD oil the default is to considers all CBD a marijuana extract. Making cannabis legal nationwide is destined to open up the gates of the burgeoning CBD market. The benefits are too great and the demand has never been higher for natural alternatives to deadly drugs.

Things are looking up for legal hemp cultivation, at least—the proposed Industrial Hemp Farming Act has bipartisan support in Congress, with many officials realizing hemp's health and economic benefits. Removing hemp forever from the list of Schedule I drugs and allowing a commercial market for hemp products could be the first step toward full acceptance by the FDA of CBD products. In the coming years, support of cannabis legalization is sure to rise as more people become educated on its many positive effects.

A Buyer's Guide
to Hemp Oil

At this point, you know the difference between CBD and THC. While they may both have therapeutic value, CBD can offer benefits without mind-altering or intoxicating effects. As an informed consumer, it is important to know the differences between the many varieties of hemp extracts and the numerous products and delivery systems that are available on the market. Under federal law, all hemp oils can be legally imported into the United Sates. Thus, with the growing availability of hemp extracts, the information out there can be very confusing when it comes to determining which hemp CBD preparations are the best—and perhaps most effective. This chapter will explain some of the confusing terms used to describe these products. We will then discuss some of the common products found on the shelves, what to look for on the labels, and in some cases, what ingredients to avoid. And just as important, you will learn how to properly store all these items.

WHAT IS HEMP OIL?

If you do any research online, it is likely you will see products referred to as hemp oil, hemp extracts, cannabidol oil, CBD oil, or even CBD hemp oil. You may also see contradictory statements as to what makes them different from one another. It can all be very confusing, so let's start with a quick refresher course. The two best-know members of the Cannabis family are marijuana and hemp. They grow as plants sprouting stalks, leaves and flowers. Each of these plants contains THC and CBD. While the marijuana variety contains more THC, from 5 to 20 percent, hemp plants contain only a fraction of this amount, not exceeding the legal limit of 0.3 percent THC (on a dry weight basis).

Normally all commercially available hemp products come from the agricultural hemp plant. It is grown around the world for its thick fibrous stalk which can be used for thousands—yes, thousands—of products. However, as useful and lucrative a hemp plant may be, the Federal government currently allows hemp to be grown for research purposes only—and only with the permission of a State's Department of Agriculture. So while the United States grows very little hemp, countries such as Canada, Holland, China, Russia, France, Spain, Hungary, Romania, Poland, Switzerland, and Chile account for a majority of the world's supply. As you will see, knowing about the seeds, genetics, and where the hemp is grown are important factors in considering a CBD product.

Oil can be extracted from any and all parts of the cannabis hemp plant. This includes its stalk, leaves, flowers, seeds, roots, and/or branches. The terms "hemp oil," "CBD oil," and "hemp extracts" are often interchanged, and often fail to clearly communicate to consumers exactly what is in the bottle being sold. The lack of standardization in this new language is expected and is due to the ambiguity surrounding the regulatory future of these products. The most important rule is not to confuse hemp seed oil with hemp extracts when you are looking for hemp CBD.

Hemp seed oil is exclusively extracted from sterilized hemp seeds, known officially as and sold as "hemp seed oil." Hemp seed oil is a nutritious energy dense source of essential fatty acids, including omega-3 ALA and omega-6 LA, yet hemp seed oils contains absolutely no THC or CBD. Hemp seed oils are sold in larger bottles, not dropper bottles, and sell for less than $20 for 16fl oz. Hemp seed oil is not what you are looking for if you are seeking hemp CBD.

Hemp oil extracts do contain CBD and THC. Depending on the environmental conditions and plant genetics used to make the extract, this results in products with a wide variation in ratios of CBD to THC, with wide ranging legal implications. The finished CBD product may therefore qualify as either a medical marijuana or agricultural hemp product that contains naturally-occurring CBD.

The easiest way to tell the difference between hemp seed oil and hemp CBD is to make absolutely sure that the Supplement facts panel on the back of the bottle reads "hemp oil (aerial plant parts)." There should be a total milligram amount of hemp oil on the first line with the second line below it listing the total cannabidiol in milligrams of CBD per serving.

"Aerial plant parts" refer to the parts of the plant the above the ground, excluding the roots. The FDA requires manufacturers to clearly list what part of the plant is being used to make the extract. Although currently only a few manufacturers label their CBD oil products in this way, consumers have the right to know exactly how much CBD they are getting per serving. It is therefore important to know the difference between hemp seed oil and hemp CBD oil extracted from the aerial plant parts, and hemp seed oil, and from which source of cannabis (hemp or marijuana) your product is made.

CBD oil or cannabidiol oil is also commercially available from marijuana, rather than hemp. These CBD products are extracted from medical drug varieties of cannabis. Remember, even CBD oil extracted from certified legal agricultural hemp that is not cultivated properly can exceed 0.3 percent THC, causing the same exact plant to be re-named and identified as marijuana. However, to be clear, CBD oil that is extracted from the marijuana flower can only be sold at dispensaries and in states with marijuana-friendly laws. This is because these products exceed the 0.3 percent THC limit and ingesting them will likely result in a high. Thus, health enthusiasts looking to avoid the intoxicating effects of THC should opt for hemp CBD oil extracts instead.

Another factor to consider when choosing a CBD oil is its refinement and concentration.

Raw Hemp CBD Oil. Raw hemp CBD oil extract is a powerful full spectrum hemp superfood. The majority of cannabinoids in raw hemp oil extracts is comprised of cannabidiolic acid, or CBDA. CBDA is the acidic precursor of CBD, which is naturally produced in the plant and contains many beneficial properties distinct from CBD. This type of CBD oil is a potent COX 2 and 15-LOX inhibitor, which means it can be used as an anti-inflammatory for systemic inflammation. Some of the issues raw CBD oil may affect are nausea, pain, acute orthopedic injuries, exercise-induced muscle soreness, rheumatoid arthritis, cancer cell migration, and autoimmune conditions. Benefits for these particular conditions have been reported with dosage for such ailments between 5 to 30 mg of CBDA dominant full spectrum hemp extract daily. Since this type of oil is the least refined, it has less of a blood-brain barrier penetration and thus is least likely to cause any effects to the central nervous system (CNS) such as somnolence.

Decarboxylated Hemp CBD Oil. When raw CBD oil is gently heated in a process known as decarboxylation, the natural CBDA content in the hemp extract is converted to activated CBD. The carboxylic acid group simply breaks off changing the structure and function of CBDA to fully activated CBD. Although many compounds existing in nature activate the endocannabinoid system, CBD is exclusively a byproduct of the decarboxylation of CBDA, meaning the near exclusive source of CBD in nature comes from heating or exposure to light in order to potentiate the chemical conversion of CBDA into activated CBD.

Hemp extracts made from certified agricultural hemp are considered full-spectrum because they contain a wide range of natural phytocannabinoids such as CBD, CBG, CBN, CBC, and traces of other cannabinoids in addition to the other natural cofactors including plant sterols, terpenes, chlorophyll, and all eight isomers of naturally-occurring vitamin E.

When activated, CBD crosses the blood-brain barrier and is reported to have profound effects in supporting nervous system health, anxiety, stress, depression, sleep, increasing insulin sensitivity, and may be used as a peripheral immunomodulator or anti-inflammatory. The dosing strategy for decarboxylated CBD Oil is always to start low (~ 2 mg of CBD) and titrate up (~ 15 mg of CBD) as needed. A protocol has been circulating for three years in the natural remedies community that recommends starting with a CBD product that delivers either 2 mg or 3mg per serving and slowly increasing the dosage of CBD to 15 mg per day over several weeks for people who are very sick, or a few days for those with more well-balanced endocannabinoid tone. The goal is to titrate the dose to minimize secondary effects like somnolence.

Optimizing and fine-tuning our endocannabinoid system may be the ultimate self-hacking modality to truly promote healing and restore balance. McPartland et al. summarized this amazing endocannabinoid system in this way: "Metaphorica, the eCB system represents a microcosm of psychoneuro-immunology or mind-body medicine." It represents a remarkable new target for a new class of compounds that defy all previous expectations of herbal extracts. You may want to combine some raw CBDA rich full spectrum hemp extract with some activated hemp CBD oil extract for additional full plant, broad spectrum synergy and support.

Gold Formula Hemp CBD Oil. Gold extracts are standardized—similar to other herbal extracts—where the plant material is distilled in a solvent-free process, concentrating CBD, other cannabinoids, fatty acids, terpenes, and naturally-occurring vitamin E. In fact, it takes approximately 10 kilograms of decarboxylated hemp CBD oil extract to yield approximately 3 kilograms of gold concentrated hemp CBD oil extract.

Concentrated CBD oil combined with lipid excipients like extra virgin olive oil have a faster onset of use because they contain more fats and fatty acids that increase the bioavailability of the fat-loving cannabinoid CBD by three fold. Gold extracts also have the highest concentration and amount of the full range of phytocannabinoids available in hemp, including ten times more of the micro-dosage of natural THC than the starting raw hemp extract itself. It's a concentrated full spectrum hemp extract at this stage that looks like a gold colored coconut fat and is now more than 50 percent fat and 25 percent CBD by volume. It's very powerful at this stage.

At this higher concentration, the mechanisms of action are through not only the endocannabinoid system, but much greater 5HT1a, TRPV, TRPA, TRPM, GABA, and PPAR receptor activation. This results in even more broad spectrum neurogenic support which may treat chronic pain, migraines, irritable bowel, fibromyalgia, cancer, addiction, treatment resistant conditions and is also beneficial in psychological health and wellness.

Consumers and practitioners have reported promising results with dosages of 3 to 60 mg daily of gold concentrated hemp CBD oil extract. Dosages of 300 mg or greater of this CBD oil extract have been suggested for very serious and chronic conditions. As always, it is key to titrate the dose slowly to maximize efficacy while minimizing undesirable side effects such as drowsiness.

For best results, especially with difficult cases, always remember to titrate the dosage. This means you should increase slowly starting with gold CBD oil drops before soft-gels or concentrates to maximize response, while minimizing secondary effects like somnolence. Try integrating gold with raw hemp CBD oil extracts for the widest possible range of phytonutrients and phytocannabonoids. This combination is targeted for the most challenging treatment resistant situations.

Finally, formal safety studies of hemp CBD oil extracts are lacking. One brand is purporting to have conducted formal toxicological safety data to support a Generally Recognized as Safe (GRAS) self conclusion for 15 mg of CBD per day from a full spectrum Gold CBD hemp oil extract. FDA acknowledges the GRAS-self-conclusion process, if done properly and if successful may offer some more regulatory clarity and distinction between hemp and Marijuana products. However, as of the publishing of this book no formal safety data on CBD has been reviewed and published in a journal since 1981.

To date, no hemp product has ever achieved anything close to GRAS status. To do so would be another monumental step in the acceptance of hemp extracts. The FDA would be in uncharted territory, as would the entire United States of America. All the evidence would point to hemp extract's safety and efficacy while none of the evidence would support prohibition or restriction of use. CBD could become both the wonder drug and nutritional ingredient of the twenty first century.

Some companies are marketing that botanical equivalents to hemp CBD can also be obtained without the use of the cannabis or hemp plant. This is patently false and may be misleading. Compounds known as *cannabimimetics* and other compounds found in extracts of ginger root, paeonia root, clove and echinacea and many other botanical sources do have some impact of the endocannabinoid system, but they are not nearly the same as CBD or THC. These clever products tout phytocannabinoids + cannabimimetics beta-caryophyllene + plant terpenes plant alkamides, however close inspection of the supplements fact panel reveals that they do not contain any CBD.

There are a number of hemp CBD brands on the market and it can be difficult to know what to look for when choosing a product that's right for you. Knowing the differences between the several types of hemp oils, the amount of CBD they deliver, and their source is the first step in choosing a product. The next thing to look for is brand transparency and understanding their supply chain process. Reading the label is also crucial in determining which type of oil you have and how much CBD, if any, is present. Lastly, quality should be a non-negotiable when it comes to making the right selection.

HOW THE OILS ARE SOLD

There is a growing number of hemp extracts now available in natural food stores, pharmacies, and online. They are available in many forms for a variety of uses. Before shopping for any specific products, you should consider which form is right for you. This includes the following:

Capsules and Softgels. These products mainly come in two forms: a capsule containing CBD oil that is spray dried onto rice flour as a green powder that is easily formulated and put into powders or capsules. Known as CBD oil capsules, they were the original full spectrum hemp derived CBD capsules in the market. Unintentionally confusing and counter intuitive these original hemp oil that was dried and powdered are still available and effective.

The state of the art delivery is ultimately soft gels made with vegetable gelatin and extra virgin olive oil to increase bioavailability by 3 fold. Softgels are available in a wide range of sizes and strengths, which should be taken as directed. The ingredients of the capsule itself may vary greatly. If formulated properly, these products contain the most precise serving sizes, in comparison to any other product.

CBD Drops and Sprays. Drops and sprays are available for full spectrum raw hemp liquid extracts, full spectrum activated hemp CBD oil extracts, and gold formula hemp CBD oil drops. Look for delicious gold formula peppermint drops sweetened with monk fruit. They tend to have the lowest amount of CBD per serving and can come in many flavors. Labels on all drops and sprays should be scrutinized, as some tinctures may contain harmful ingredients. Because drops and sprays are easy to manufacture and can be made at home, the quality of the product may be compromised. To avoid this, it is imperative to read the supplement facts panel and ask for a Certificate of Analysis (COA). The solution is to be taken orally, and normally sublingually—under the tongue.

Balms. The least invasive of all CBD products, topical balms are widely available and are normally applied to the skin. They may also be blended with other herbs and oils. While some products may be marketed as "transdermal," meaning absorbed through the skin, the science behind this kind of rub has not yet been fine-tuned, and is considered a drug delivery system by FDA. The commercially available raw and gold balms can only be absorbed on the surface of the skin, similar to most lotions. Balms made with raw hemp oil extracts are reported to help with dry, itchy and flaky skin, even eczema and psoriasis.

Concentrates. This form is the most pure and natural way to administer any hemp product. They are pure concentrates free of any other added carrier oil or ingredient. Look for products that list other ingredients as "none" on the supplement facts panel to make sure it's a pure hemp extract concentrate. As mentioned in the previous section, there are many forms of hemp oil. Always pay attention to which type of oil is desired, and make sure the label reflects that oil, whether it be sourced from marijuana or from certified agricultural hemp.

Vaporizers. These can refer to two types of inhalers: concentrate vaporizers and e-liquid vaporizers. Concentrate vaporizers are specifically designed to vaporize pure CBD concentrates that contain no added ingredients. Some CBD concentrates come prefilled in cartridges that attach to a vaporizer pen. There are also some specifically designed for the oil to be put directly onto the device for vaporization as well.

E-liquid CBD is also available in cartridge form. However, these cartridges usually contain other ingredients, mainly propylene glycol (PEG) or vegetable glycerin (VG). A less common ingredient that may also be used is polyethylene terephthalate resin (PET). Most of the time CBD, products containing PEG or PET should be avoided unless they are being used to quit or reduce combustion cigarette smoking or smokeless tobacco addiction. Risk reward benefits must always be carefully measured. Purified CBD vape shows tremendous promise for harm reduction and helping people break the crippling addiction to nicotine.

In addition to the products listed above, there are a number of other forms CBD comes in that you may wish to know more about. See inset on page 40 for details. While it's good to find a product that you are comfortable using, there are a number of important factors to consider when evaluating one product from another. The next section will provide you with some important things to keep in mind when making your selection.

HOW THE OILS ARE EXTRACTED

There are several ways to draw the oil out of the hemp plant. The three which are most popular are the carbon dioxide method, the ethanol-based method, and the cold pressing method (which is typically only used for hemp seed oil). When any of these extraction methods use hemp that has been grown to high standards, the results should be clean hemp oil.

Cold Pressing. Cold pressing is used when extracting oil from hemp seeds Here, the seeds, either whole or ground down, are put into a press where the oil is pressed out of the seeds. The heat created by friction should not exceed 120° F. This extraction method should only be used to extract oil from hemp seeds and is not helpful in producing oil high in cannabinoids, including

CBD. This method is not likely to filter out any chemical impurities that the hemp seeds may contain.

Carbon Dioxide (CO2) Method. This method is one of the most popular, safe, and environmentally friendly extraction methods. It is the current standard for food and herbal supplements in the industry, where it is used for a variety of products, ranging from essential oils to decaffeinated coffee.

The hemp is placed under pressure with the carbon dioxide (CO2) in order to extract the oils from the plant. After this process is complete, the CO2 and the extract are moved from the pressure vessel to another location. In subcritical extraction, the CO2 is placed at lower temperatures, and after passing through the extraction vessel, it is moved to an evaporator, where the CO2 can return to a gas form and be released back into the atmosphere to be recycled. When supercritical CO2 is used, the CO2 is placed at higher temperatures, then separated from the extract after it goes through the extraction vessel. The extract then settles at lower temperatures. Once the CO2 has cooled, it can be re-compressed and recycled, or released back into the atmosphere. Ideally, look for hemp that is extracted using the Carbon Dioxide (CO2) method.

Solvent-based Extraction Method. In this process, the hemp sections are submerged into a liquid solvent, such as ethanol, butane, or a combination of CO2 and another solvent (which is less common). In this method, the hemp plant and solvent of choice are combined together and placed into the separation equipment.

There are two ways this can be done: One way is to put the solvent and

A World of CBD Products

Today, there is a wide variety of CBD products available. As a customer it is important to check the source of the CBD and the amount of CBD in the product, perform potency testing to make sure the label meets claims, and check that the other ingredients that are present.

- CBD Apple Cider Vinegar
- CBD Chocolate Bars
- CBD Coconut Oil
- CBD Gum
- CBD Gummy Candies
- CBD Lozenges
- CBD Teas and Drinks
- CBD Water Soluble
- Isolated CBD Crystalline
- Natural Hemp and Propolis Healing Salve

plant material into an auger conveyor, and separate the plant material from the extract. Another way is to spray the solvent of choice on the hemp as it enters the separation equipment, such as a centrifugal separator or belt press. In both cases, the "latency period" (the time between the combination of the solvent and the material, and the separation of the two) is a timed process where the temperature must be monitored to stay at cooler temperatures. After which, the extract and the solvent are quickly separated from each other. This process is not particularly harmful, but if not done properly the resulting oil may have some residual solvents present.

Solvents are used to convert cannabis or hemp that may not be fresh enough or clean enough to be extracted with cold pressing or carbon dioxide CO_2. They offer the possibility to extract commercially salable cannabinoids, even if the plant material is starting to rot and decompose. Even when producing 100 percent pure and natural isolated cannabinoids, solvent extraction is required.

Solvent extraction, especially butane, can produce widely coveted medical marijuana extracts, known as butane hash oil. These products are only legally sold in marijuana dispensaries.

If the solvent-based extraction method is utilized with the intention of making full spectrum agricultural hemp CBD oil extracts, insist on seeing third party test results proving the absence of any residual solvents, such as pentane and butane.

Most often, solvent extraction is used to make pure CBD crystals known as isolates. Isolates are just that, isolated CBD devoid of nearly all cofactors and natural plant buffers. Isolates are the exact opposite of full spectrum hemp oil CBD extracts. They are closer to drugs and are not traditionally considered the kind of natural extract one would find in a health food store.

Based on the intellectual property rights surrounding pure CBD in addition to definitions of what technically differentiates a drug from a natural extract, isolated CBD crystals may end up only being available behind a pharmacy counter.

The bigger question with isolated CBD crystals is, are they actually synthetic or are the crystals natural? Properly made natural isolated CBD crystals can and fetch upwards of 50,000 per kilo for 99 percent pure CBD isolate.

Nanotechnology Delivery. Hemp seed oil or hemp CBD oil extracts produced with cold pressing, carbon dioxide (CO_2) method and even solvent-based extraction methods, may undergo additional processing with the promise of increased absorption or bioavailability. They can be sold under the names CBD water, water soluble CBD, liposomal, nanoemulsified or nanotechnology. These delivery systems may increase bioavailability in laboratory cell models and even in limited human studies. However, is it proof that we need less of these forms of CBD to get identical results from higher milligram amounts?

Products that claim to be 5 times more bioavailable than natural hemp CBD oil extracts, for example, infer that only 2mg of enhanced absorption water soluble CBD or liposomal CBD will deliver the exact same effect as 10 mg of CBD from hemp oil extract. These claims are not proven to be accurate and are currently premature.

Remember that these delivery systems reduce the size of the droplet with the intent of driving the CBD deeper into tissues and through the body. If the starting material used is contaminated, even with non-detectable levels of toxins, aflatoxins, mold, fungus, heavy metals, solvents or worse synthetic CBD or CBD like analogs, the unknowns may outweigh perceived advantage over hemp extracts.

Thus it's important to note that bioavailability and enhanced absorption claims of cannabinoids exceed the scientific data and may be more marketing than science.

THE GOOD, THE BAD, AND THE UGLY

Because of the gray area in which hemp products exist in the marketplace, by making sure you find the right product, you can reap the maximum benefits from this magnificent plant. The following points are essential to know when considering what product to buy.

Origin of the Products

In the beginning of this chapter, we talked about the many countries throughout the world that now produce hemp. While growing hemp may be good for these countries' economies, the problem for consumers using a hemp product is the uncertainty of what other unhealthful substances the plant may contain. In many of these hemp-growing nations, the rules for the use of dangerous pesticides and herbicides in growing these crops are lax or not stringently enforced. So while the original intent for growing these crops may not be for human consumption, many of these plants may find their way to secondary marketplaces that are specifically aimed at the health and beauty market.

Likewise, many quality manufacturers are committed to using certified hemp cultivars that are also used in the production of food grade hemp products. These food grade varieties of hemp are cultivated as agricultural crops and will prove to be ideal source of CBD.

In addition, the hemp plant is considered a "bioaccumulator." What this means is that the plant has the ability to absorb heavy metals and other chemical wastes found in the soil it grows in. Again, where the hemp is grown for non-human consumption that should not be a problem; however, you may be putting yourself at risk by not knowing the origin of the hemp in the product you may be using.

To avoid this problem, it is important to ask the manufacturer for documentation on their hemp sourcing. Again, while the original purpose for growing hemp in most other countries was for fiber, there are varieties that are grown in a manner that is more targeted for nutrition and medical use. Typically any manufacturer committed to quality and safety will gladly share this data with its consumers upon request. Knowing these facts can be illuminating. However, the savvy and discerning consumer knows that growing location or even certification fails to ensure toxicological safety at the recommended daily intake.

Hemp, like all plants, reflects the condition of its environment. The cleaner the environment, the cleaner the plant, the cleaner the product is in a logical refrain. Considering most consumers take between 5 to 15 mg of CBD per day from hemp CBD oil extracts, knowing that the ingested extract is proven fit for daily human consumption is the definitive test of safety.

According to a recent safety review published in *Cannabis and Cannabinoid Research*, "Several aspects of a toxicological evaluation of a compound such as genotoxicity studies and research evaluating CBD effect on hormones are still scarce. Especially, chronic studies on CBD's effect on, for example, genotoxicity and the immune system, are still missing." They are very safe and non-toxic in humans. However, satisfying FDA's requirement of toxicological studies to investigate the safety of oral consumption of a new product to support a GRAS self-conclusion is a different process than gaining organic certification, third party testing, or even human clinical trials with CBD.

These formal toxicology studies are required by law to introduce a new "food" into the human food supply. Hemp is ancient and hemp products have proven to be safe, yet hemp extracts are concentrated from whatever plant was used. The variables for contamination and exposure are troubling considering how much CBD will be required to meet the overwhelming demand.

Products that differentiate themselves with concerted evidence based safety assessments required to obtain Generally Recognized as Safe Status (GRAS) must be conducted at a GLP, FDA, OECD, EU, EC compliant toxicology lab. The studies included: AMES bacterial reverse mutation study (mutagenicity), chromosomal aberration study (clastogenicity), in vivo mouse micronucleus study (genotoxicity), 14-day repeated dose oral toxicity study in rats, and a ninety day repeated dose toxicity study in rats. The substance needs to be proven not to be mutagenic, clastogenic, or genotoxic. The pivotal studies to support a GRAS self-conclusion or an FDA GRAS Notification are the three genotoxicity studies and the ninety day study. A NOAEL (no observed adverse effect level) must be established from the ninety day study. This battery of toxicological studies must be written in the form of a manuscript and submitted to the peer-reviewed academic journal that specializes in toxicology.

An established formula is to apply a 100-fold safety factor to determine if the serving size on the product is proven to be GRAS for the indented results. Look for a company's rating on the internet or through the Better Business Bureau (see Resource Section on page 113). You can also contact the company directly to ask questions or for actual copies of a certified organic license. While this is not always an easy task, it will be worth the effort. Several hemp seed oil and hemp foods manufacturers have attained certified organic status. Some hemp growers are claiming to be growing on organically certified land. However, none of the hemp CBD oil extracts themselves are truly "Certified Organic," even if the hemp is grown in complete accordance with all organic farming standards.

You may see the word "natural" on the label as well. Unfortunately, there is no real criteria for the use of the word. While it may refer to the fact that none of the ingredients in the product have been produced synthetically, it does not indicate that the hemp plant used has been certified organic. Without a legal definition, the word "natural" may simply be a marketing ploy to get your attention.

Other Active Ingredients

As more and more hemp products are made available, different manufacturers will add various other ingredients to their products. For example, today you will find not only plain CBD oils, but you will also find CBD tinctures, drops and sprays CBD chocolate and gummies, Gold CBD in extra-virgin olive oil—the list goes on. These products are not pure CBD oil products, but formulations that contain CBD oil, mixed in carrier oils or other ingredients.

The most important thing to look out for in these particular products is the quality of the other ingredients, and if the CBD claim on the product matches the content in the actual formula. Have any additives been added for color enhancement or to make the product last longer? What chemicals or natural ingredients have been mixed in to make the product smell better? Does the company offer testing results for the potency of their products?

While the hemp oil may not pose a problem in and of itself, another ingredient may cause an allergic reaction or may be problematic when taken with a specific prescription drug. It is therefore very important to carefully look at the label to see what ingredients the product contains. If you have questions about any of the ingredients in a product, ask a pharmacist or healthcare professional for help to determine the safety of a product you are not sure about.

What is the Shelf Life of Hemp Oil Extracts?

As a rule of thumb, hemp CBD extracts will normally last in an unopened airtight bottle from twelve to eighteen months from the time of its manufacture. Once opened, it can last for another twelve months as long as it is stored in a dark bottle, kept in a cool area, and away from light. While it is most common to place opened bottles in the refrigerator, for some CBD products this is not recommended. As always, read the labels or contact the company if you are unsure of how to store your product.

Like any essential fatty oil, over a long period of time hemp oil will degrade, diminishing its therapeutic properties. It will also turn rancid when exposed to oxygen, light, and heat. Should the oil become oxidized, it would usually change to a darker color and give off an acrid odor, as though something was burning. It's important to throw out any oils that you believe have expired. The simplest way to avoid the possibility of the oil becoming rancid is to purchase one to three months' worth of oils at a time.

POTENCY

All hemp oil CBD extract potency differs from one product to another. The level of potency is subject to several manufacturing factors:

- The specific part or parts of the hemp plant used.

- The extraction process used to draw out the oil.

- The way the extracted oil may be concentrated.

- The amount of other ingredients added to the extracted oil.

- The ability for the manufacturer to standardize their oil production.

As mentioned earlier, any company that is properly manufacturing CBD products will have potency results from an independent testing lab, and may also have results from their own laboratory analysis. Products such as sprays and drops (tinctures) will typically have lower concentrations of CBD per serving, because the oil is mixed in with other ingredients.

Some labels may claim to contain 1000 mg CBD in an entire bottle of product, but still only deliver as little as 1 mg per serving. Softgels and capsules are also mixed with other ingredients, but can contain up to 30 mg per softgel/capsule, and even more if made with isolated CBD crystals. Concentrated natural form, without any other ingredients, will typically have the highest milligram amount per serving.

If the milligram amount of CBD is not printed on the label it may confuse the consumer interested in how much CBD is in the bottle. Unfortunately, this is a regulatory tactic taken by uneducated or unscrupulous marketers of CBD products. With the hope of avoiding DEA, FDA, or DOJ enforcement, most sellers of hemp extracts today have elected to remove all references to cannabidiol CBD and the more potent peripheral anti-inflammatory cannabidiolic acid CBDA found in raw hemp oil extracts. Even sellers who do make ultra-high-quality food grade hemp extracts that are safe and effective may elect to eliminate any mention of CBD on the label until the Food and Drug Administration has an official position.

Just because the brand decides not to call out the cannabidiol (CBD) in the supplement facts panel does not mean that it's an inferior hemp extract. The only way to ensure the potency of the product is as stated on the label, is to acquire test results ideally from the manufacturer's in-house laboratory, along with corroborating third party testing for purity and potency from an accredited and respected independent laboratory.

The most valid and cutting critique of the burgeoning hemp extract industry are failed label claims. The majority of available CBD products today do not deliver the amount of CBD that is advertised. The FDA has the ability to liquidate a seller in the market who claims 15 mg per serving when it only contains 5 mg.

The analytical testing issue is further complicated one again because of the regulatory ambiguity of the cannabis hemp plant itself. This ambiguity is preventing the acceptance of cannabinoid testing standards, resulting in widely noted variation in cannabinoid content, even among accredited and respected laboratories. Groups like Consumer Lab have announced mass testing of CBD oil products and from existing data sets from laboratories that routinely test hundreds of brands. They have been tracking a 80 percent failure rate, meaning only 20 percent of the products tested actually contained what the consumer thought they were buying and more importantly getting for their health. In the end, no matter what it is, you only need answer one simple question? Is hemp CBD oil working for you?

ARE THEY WORKING?

If you are taking a CBD oil to treat a particular health problem, it is important to consult a healthcare professional. The bottom line is that you want the product to work, and that cannot always be determined without professional guidance. As you will see in Part 2 of this book, there are many serious disorders that CBD has been shown to reduce in severity and even alleviate. There have been numerous medical studies published that have shown the effectiveness of CBD on many health issues.

However, it is important to point out that while CBD has proven to be effective in many cases, it may not work for everyone in the same way. First, our bodies are all different—from our unique DNA to the biochemistry that is us. This can make a big difference in outcome. Secondly, differing results can also stem from the specific product you are using to the amount you are taking. Therefore, before taking any CBD products to treat a health problem, it is important to consult a healthcare professional.

Once you are using CBD for any given problem, however, the fact is, you would also be the best judge to see if it is working. Over time, if it seems not to be helping, make sure that the oil you are using is the right oil. Consider changing the product to another brand. If you do not see or feel any positive changes over time, feel free to discontinue its use. Do not be afraid to look for other options that may provide potential relief.

CONCLUSION

"Let the buyer beware" is an important phrase to keep in mind when looking for most any products. As someone who may be trying to overcome a health issue, this phrase is doubly important. Today, there are many unsubstantiated claims floating around the internet—many designed to sell products. Unfortunately, hype is no substitute for facts. As a customer looking for the best product, your job is to become a smart consumer. By taking the time to learn the facts, you will be in a better position to ask the right questions and make informed decisions. Hopefully this chapter will help you on your journey to a healthier you.

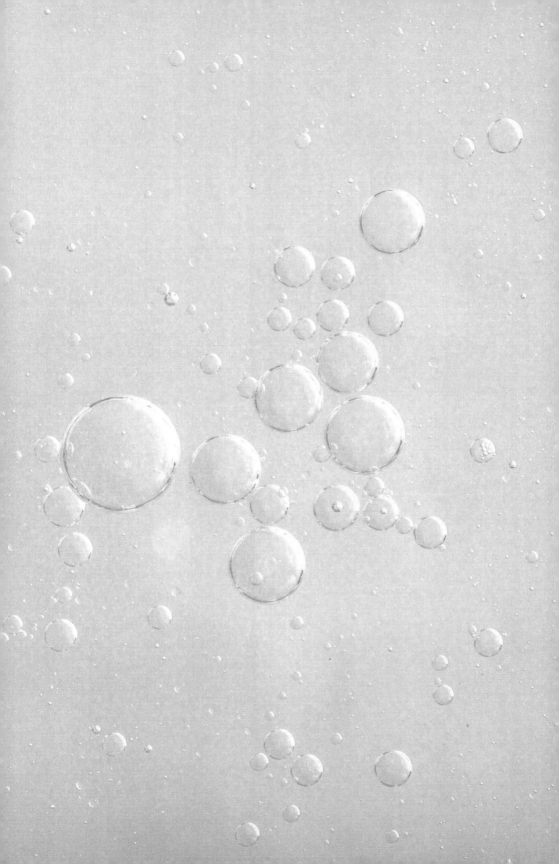

PART TWO

Healing With Hemp CBD Oil

An Alphabetical Guide to Using Cannabinoid & Hemp CBD Oil

Hemp oil consists of high-CBD and low-THC hemp. Unlike medical marijuana products, which are highly concentrated in THC, hemp oil contains only trace amounts, making it a safer product that provides important health benefits without the psychoactive effects. It is available in a number of concentrations and forms, such as liquid hemp oil; concentrate balms; vapor from vaporizers; easy to take and convenient vegetarian softgels capsules, sublingual tinctures, drops or sprays with extra virgin olive oil; even edibles in the form of candy. Topical CBD balms may also be effective for acne. Treatment resistant skin conditions may require much higher concentrations and in this application, isolated CBD crystals may prove to be ideal.

Gold full spectrum hemp extracts have also been reported to be very effective and may appeal more to the natural and organic shopper looking to avoid solvents. High quality gold concentrates list other ingredients on the back of the supplement facts panel as NONE, meaning it's 100 percent hemp extract. Make sure when using concentrated hemp extracts topically to avoid your eyes. For internal inflammation and the role of cannabinoids on flora skin connection Take approximately 5 to 15 mg of CBD daily internally in addition to topical washing or applications. Hemp seed oil with omega 3 ALA in addition to marine omega 3 EPA and DHA.

AD

See **ALZHEIMER'S DISEASE.**

ADDICTION, OPIATE

Opiate addiction is a serious problem in the United States today. Opiates include a vast assortment of drugs, ranging from legal drugs such as fentanyl, codeine, and morphine, to illegal drugs such as heroin and opium. Over a period of time people become physically reliant on these drugs. This addiction can occur if the drugs are prescribed by a doctor or if they are being used illegally.

Symptoms

An indication of an opiate addiction is when an individual continues using even when they are aware that there are negative consequences. Some physical signs of this addiction are characterized by:

- Constipation
- Constricted pupils
- Drowsiness/marked sedation
- Elation
- Euphoria
- Loss of consciousness
- Mood swings
- Noticeable confusion

Triggers

What may trigger drug use and/or abuse for one individual may be different for someone else. However, the following are triggers that are common to most people:

- Anxiety
- Chronic illness
- Chronic pain
- Depression
- Frustration
- Rejection
- Stress

Conventional Treatment/Side Effects

There are now drugs available to treat opiate addictions. They are categorized as *agonists* and *partial agonists,* which act like opiates but are safer and less addictive, and *antagonists,* which block the addictive effects of opiates. But they are not without side effects. Agonists such as methadone, hydrocodone bitartrate, and oxycodone hydrochloride may have similar side effects as heroin and may trigger depressed breathing. Buprenorphine, a partial agonist, may cause nausea and constipation. Naltrexone, an antagonist, may block pain relief if you are using an opiate medication for pain.

CBD and Hemp Oil

Research has shown that CBD has "a very low abuse potential and inhibits drug-seeking behavior." In an animal study, researchers found that the effects of CBD lasted as long as two weeks after it was administered, while methadone needed to be administered daily to be effective. The potential of CBD's effect on decreasing the opiate addiction "by lowering its overall effect on the central nervous system" was also cited in the study.

In 2017, there were ninety-one deaths from opiate overdose a day in the United States. CBD is a plant, not a man-made drug. It's not addictive, and has minimal side effects at recommended doses. As stated in a 2015 report by the Partnership for Drug-Free Kids, "there are hundreds of people in Massachusetts being treated with medical pot in order to control their addiction to opioids. There have been so many opiate-linked deaths in the state that doctors are getting patients on to non-addictive cannabis [CBD] as much as they can to stop more fatalities from occurring."

Dr. Dustin Sulak, the founder and director of Integr8 Health stated: " In addition to keeping people in treatment, replacing and reducing the opioids, improving the pain relief that opioids provide, and preventing opioid dose escalation and tolerance, cannabis can also treat the symptoms of opioid withdrawal: nausea, vomiting, diarrhea, abdominal cramping, muscle spasms, anxiety, agitation, restlessness, insomnia, and also minor symptoms like runny nose and sweating."

How to Use: Recommended dosage is 15 to 45 mg multiple times daily. For very difficult cases, THC may also be helpful for patients who can tolerate it. Check with health care provider before using THC.

CBDA, CBD, THC and other cannabinoids represent a new group of natural anti-addiction agents. CBD is currently being developed as a drug to treat smokeless tobacco addiction. The initial findings are remarkable and the future for these natural plant-based signaling molecules or extracts to address multiple forms of addiction should be considered.

ADHD

See **ATTENTION DEFICIT HYPERACTIVITY DISORDER.**

AGE-RELATED MACULAR DEGENERATION

Age-related macular degeneration (AMD) generally impacts older adults, over the age of 60. It is a medical disease affecting the eye, generating a loss of vision in the macula (the center of the visual field) because of damage that has occurred to the retina. There are two forms of AMD:

1. *Dry AMD:* This form develops from atrophy to the retinal pigment epithelial layer below the retina.

2. *Wet AMD:* This form occurs due to abnormal blood vessel growth causing damaging and rapid vision loss if not treated.

Symptoms

You may not experience any symptoms in the early stages of AMD; however, the first sign of the condition may be characterized by a gradual or sudden change in the quality of your vision. Other symptoms may include:

- Changes in perception of color, in rare cases
- Dark, blurry areas
- Loss of central vision
- Whiteout in the center of your vision

Triggers

The condition may be inherited. If a family member has been diagnosed with macular degeneration, you may run a higher risk of developing the condition. Other triggers include:

- Diet
- High blood pressure
- High cholesterol
- Inactivity
- Lighter eye color
- Obesity
- Smoking

Conventional Treatment/Side Effects

Although there is no cure for this disease, drugs like Lucentis and Avastin have been used to slow or prevent increased loss of vision. Injections in the eye, such as Macugen and Eylea, may also be prescribed to slow down the loss of vision.

Even though these treatments have been FDA-approved for treating AMD, there may be possible serious side effects associated with their use, such as:

- Bleeding (bloodshot eye) or discharge from the eye
- Eye infections
- Eye pain, redness
- Flashes of light or floaters
- Retinal detachment
- Sensitivity to light
- Swelling around the eyes
- Swelling of the cornea
- Vision problems

In addition to the use of drugs as a treatment, laser surgery is another option.

CBD and Hemp Oil

In Chapter 2, you were introduced to the endocannabinoid system, which is comprised of a number of cannabinoid receptors that impact our body's physiological processes. Each of these receptors are present in the cells of our body, including the eyes, and have different effects on the tissues.

Correlations have been cited between the healing power of CBD and workings of age-related macular degeneration. In a Finnish study published in the journal *Pharmacology & Therapeutics* in 2002, the researchers observed that the eye has cannabinoid receptors. The study concluded that "smoking cannabis directly was found to lower intraocular pressure in glaucoma patients."

CB1 receptors in the endocannabinoid system affect the area of the eye that is responsible for eye pressure. CB2 receptors affect the retina and the cornea. It is probable that these molecules can positively affect these particular tissues, and conceivably, the progression of AMD. More research is needed to show details of these receptors and how the tissues react to these molecules.

Cannabinoids have been shown to help AMD symptoms. Research has cited that cannabinoids:

- Are anti-inflammatory for the retina area
- Are neuro-protective
- Are anti-angiogenesis
- Have anti-aging properties
- Inhibit VEGF growth (vascular endothelial growth factor), the growth of new blood vessels
- Lowers blood pressure
- Protects retina cells
- Reduce ocular pressure

How to Use: Recommended dosage is 3 to 30. THC may also be needed in some cases, provided the patient can tolerate THC. If not, a larger dose of

CBD may be effective, up to 120 mg per day. Hemp seed oil with omega 3 ALA in addition to marine omega 3 EPA and DHA may enhance benefits.

If you are trying an enhanced delivery system form of CBD and not achieving the desired results, then take the same milligram serving from a hemp extract that lists the milligram amount of CBD on the label. Analytical purity and potency results that are validated by non-negotiable third party independent results corroborate precisely how much CBD per serving you are really getting.

ALZHEIMER'S DISEASE

Alzheimer's disease is a progressive brain disorder that gradually brings about the destruction of large numbers of nerve cells in the brain. It slowly impairs memory and thinking skills and eventually leads to an inability to carry out simple tasks. Medical experts suggest that over 5 million Americans may have been diagnosed with Alzheimer's disease in the U.S. At the present time it is ranked as the sixth leading cause of death.

Symptoms

In the beginning, the only symptom that may be noticeable is forgetfulness, confusion, or difficulty organizing your thoughts. However, as the disease progresses the changes in the brain may lead to:

- Behavior changes
- Confusion with time
- Changes in mood
- Difficulty forming judgments and making decisions
- Difficulty planning
- Difficulty carrying out and completing familiar tasks
- Difficulty thinking and reasoning
- Disruptive memory loss
- Personality changes
- Problems speaking
- Withdrawal from social interest

Triggers

Scientists still don't have a completely clear understanding of what causes Alzheimer's disease in most people, however they believe that genetics, lifestyle, and environmental factors come into play. Over time these elements may affect the brain. Evidence suggests many theories that may put you at risk for developing Alzheimer's, including the following factors:

- Age
- Diabetes, type 2
- Diet
- Drugs
- Exposure to toxic substances
- Genetics
- Head injury
- High blood pressure
- High cholesterol level
- Lack of exercise
- Obesity
- Sleep deprivation
- Smoking

Conventional Treatment/Side Effects

Currently, the two medications most commonly prescribed as a treatment for Alzheimer's are cholinesterase inhibitors and memantine. The effectiveness of these drugs differ from person to person.

Cholinesterase inhibitors and memantine drugs may slow down the progression of the disease, but not without side effects. The cholinesterase inhibitors may cause nausea, vomiting, appetite loss, or frequent bowel movements; in particular, the drug donepezil has been associated with seizures. Memantine drugs may result in headaches, constipation, confusion and dizziness.

Scientists are searching to find new treatments because the current treatments mask the symptoms, but do not treat the underlying disease. In 2006, *The New York Times* cited a study done by *The New England Journal of Medicine* which indicated that "drugs most commonly used to soothe agitation and aggression in people with Alzheimer's disease are no more effective than placebos for most patients, and put them at risk of serious side effects, including confusion, sleepiness, and Parkinson's disease-like symptoms, researchers are reporting today."

There is no cure, prevention, or treatment to slow the advancement of Alzheimer's.

CBD and Hemp Oil

The starting point for change to evolve in the medical treatment of Alzheimer's is the acknowledgement that today's treatments are not safe or effective, and although they may reduce symptoms, the conventional drug cannot reverse or slow down the progression of the disease. CBD has been shown to reverse cognitive deficits of Alzheimer's transgenic mice. A study cited in a 2014 issue of the *Journal of Alzheimer's Disease* was the earliest to give evidence of CBD's ability to avert the occurrence of a social recognition deficit in AD transgenic mice. According to the study, "control and Alzhemier's transgenic mice were treated orally from 2.5 months of age with CBD (20 mg/kg) daily for 8 months. Mice were then assessed in the social preference test, elevated plus maze, and fear conditioning paradigms, before cortical and hippocampal tissues were analyzed for amyloid load, oxidative damage, cholesterol, phytosterols, and inflammation. [The researchers] found that AβPP × PS1 mice developed a social recognition deficit, which was prevented by CBD treatment." The data gives [them] initial evidence that CBD may be viable as a preventative treatment for Alzhemier's symptoms such as social withdrawal and facial recognition.

Research has shown that CBD aides in neurogenesis, the generation of new neurons in the hippocampus area of the brain. It is in this part of the brain where memory is formed, organized, and stored. This is crucial since neurons play an important role in the transmission of messages within the brain as well as throughout the nervous system. CBD can help to prevent the formation of Alzheimer's plaques in the brain.

Dr. David Schubert, a professor at the Salk Institute, studied the effects of cannabinoids on Alzheimer's treatment. His findings show that CBD may reduce the amount of beta-amyloid, a protein fragment commonly thought to cause the neurodegenerative disease, in the brain. He stated: "Although other studies have offered evidence that cannabinoids might be neuroprotective against the symptoms of Alzheimer's, we believe our study is the first to demonstrate that cannabinoids affect both inflammation and amyloid beta accumulation in nerve cells."

How to Use: Recommended dosage is 330 mg. Some reports suggest marijuana has been shown to slow and even reverse Alzheimer's in rats. THC may be effective, if tolerated. Check with health care provider before using cannabis or THC products. Taking small amounts of CBD when feelings of stress and anxiety are high have also been reported. Hemp seed oil with omega 3 ALA in addition to marine omega 3 EPA and DHA may enhance benefits.

AMD

See **AGE-RELATED MACULAR DEGENERATION.**

ANXIETY DISORDERS

The occasional occurrence of anxiety is a normal part of life. However, when it occurs more frequently and causes such distress that it restricts your ability to function and gets in the way of leading a normal life, anxiety can become disabling and a serious mental disorder. Anxiety can present itself in various ways, such as panic attacks, phobias, and social fears. It has been established that anxiety and related disorders affect about 40 million adults age eighteen and older.

Symptoms

Anxiety disorders are characterized by symptoms that appear suddenly and become so chronic that they disrupt our daily lives. These symptoms include:

- Chest pain
- Feeling of choking
- Heart palpitations
- Inability to relax
- Muscle tension
- Poor concentration
- Sweating
- Upset stomach

Triggers

A number of factors may trigger anxiety. The causes or risk factors for generalized anxiety disorders (GAD) may include:

- Caffeine
- Family history of anxiety
- Family illnesses
- Fears
- Illnesses
- Stressful situations, severe or long-lasting

Conventional Treatment/Side Effects

Most physicians prescribe selective serotonin reuptake inhibitors (SSRIs) or serotonin norepinephrine reuptake inhibitors (SNRIs) as treatment for anxiety disorders. Some feel that these medications should be supplemented with cognitive-behavioral therapy (CBT) to be most effective. Prescription anxiety mediations such as SSRIs may result in weight gain, insomnia, and sexual dysfunction. Antidepressants have proven to increase the risk of suicide in adolescents up to twenty-four years of age.

CBD and Hemp Oil

Evidence gathered from animal studies and human experimental, clinical, and epidemiological studies point to elements in CBD that may be favorable in treating various anxiety-related conditions, including:

- Depression
- Obsessive Compulsive Disorder
- Panic disorders
- Post-Traumatic Stress
- Social fears (phobia)

Like SSRIs, CBD may also target the serotonin system by helping the brain cells transmit more serotonin signals, which help to alleviate anxiety and heighten mood.

In an animal study, Spanish researchers studied the effects of 3 to 45 mg of CBD daily. Hemp seed oil with omega 3 ALA in addition to marine omega 3 EPA and DHA may enhance benefits.

APPETITE LOSS

A decreased or loss of appetite occurs when you have a reduced desire to eat and dulled taste buds. While a healthy appetite is characteristic of positive health, loss of appetite may be a sign of a number of problems.

Symptoms

The primary symptoms associated with a loss of appetite are malnutrition and unintentional weight loss. Fatigue and loss of appetite combined leads to dizziness, fainting, blurry vision, lethargy, and a racing heartbeat. If left untreated, these conditions may become serious.

Triggers

A variety of conditions or diseases may lead to a loss of appetite. It can be triggered by physical illness or mental illness. Feelings of grief, depression, and anxiety can also stifle the appetite. Some of the conditions may be serious, such as certain cancers, chronic liver disease, kidney failure, thyroid disorders, infection, or dementia. Appetite loss is also a potential side effect of a number of medications, including antidepressants and antibiotics.

Conventional Treatment/Side Effects

Most commonly prescribed drugs for appetite loss include antiemetics, which are typically recommended for nausea and vomiting, and antihistamines. Although these medications enhance the appetite, they generally cause a wide range of negative side effects.

CBD and Hemp Oil

Although research into the benefits of CBD and appetite loss is still in the early stages, one of the significant benefits researchers have found is the use of CBD as a digestive aid. Studies suggest that cannabinoid receptors play a crucial role in controlling eating behavior. When CBD binds to C1 receptors, it stimulates the appetite while easing nausea and vomiting. This has been especially helpful for treating patients undergoing chemotherapy, as well as other serious diseases. Cannabinoids may also assist in dealing with emotional disorders, which affects one's interest in food.

How to Use: According to the Mayo Clinic, the suggested dosage to increase appetite in cancer patients is 2.5 milligrams of THC by mouth with or without 1 mg of CBD for six weeks. As the dosage of CBD differs for each person, it is best to start small and gradually increase until you experience the desired result. Raw CBDA rich hemp extracts may also be effective for increasing appetite. It is recommended to take anywhere from one to six servings (capsules or soft gels) daily. Cannabis and THC are known to enhance appetite, however use should be monitored by an experienced physician. Hemp seed oil with omega 3 ALA in addition to marine omega 3 EPA and DHA may enhance benefits.

ARTHRITIS

Arthritis is an inflammatory condition that can affect one or multiple joints. It occurs when the immune system begins to attack healthy joints. Although there are many different types of arthritis, the three most common are osteoarthritis, rheumatoid arthritis, and psoriatic arthritis. Osteoarthritis occurs most often and is characterized by the wear and tear of overused joints; rheumatoid arthritis materializes when the immune system strikes parts of the body causing inflammation and damage to the joints; and psoriatic arthritis is a condition defined by an inflammation of the skin and joints.

Symptoms

Commonly, the symptoms and signs are associated with the joints. Depending on the kind of arthritis you have, you may experience:

- Decreased range of motion
- Muscle and joint pain
- Fatigue
- Stiffness
- Joint redness and warmth
- Swelling

Most types of arthritis are triggered by a combination of varied factors.

Triggers

Again, the cause of arthritis pain depends on the type or form of arthritis you have. There is no single cause for the hundreds of kinds of arthritis. Common factors that may be potential causes may include:

- Abdominal pain
- Fatigue

- Genetics
- Immune system dysfunction
- Infection

- Injury

- Stress

Conventional Treatment/Side Effects

Nonsteroidal Anti-inflammatory Drugs (NSAIDs) may aid in alleviating pain and inflammation in the various kinds of arthritis, but they are associated with a number of side effects, including stomach bleeding. They also pose the risk of cardiovascular problems, such as heart attack and stroke.

Acetaminophen, such as Tylenol, has anti-pyretic (anti-fever) properties and relieves arthritis pain as well. However, it can trigger liver and kidney problems. Steroids may also decrease inflammation, but they increase the risk of infection and cataracts and may result in weakened bones. Disease-modifying anti-rheumatic drugs (DMARDs) decelerate—but do not reverse—joint damage, which can bring about side effects, such as increased risk of serious infection.

CBD and Hemp Oil

In a rodent study, researchers discovered that CBD was effective in lessening inflammation and pain associated with arthritis, leading them to the conclusion that CBD has potential in treating chronic pain. In this study, the researchers observed both inflammatory and neuropathic pain.

Doctors have cited that cannabinoid oil plays a role in the treatment of all types of arthritis. In a study conducted in 2006, patients suffering from rheumatoid arthritis who used cannabinoid oil for a period of 5 weeks experienced less pain and reduced inflammation.

A 2013 study published in *Rheumatology* found that both CBD and THC engage with CB2 receptors and that "CBD increases the amount of endocannabiniods in the body. By directly engaging with the endocannabinoid system, cannabis taps into the body's own system of self-repair. The herb calms inflammation and reigns in the immune system, giving your nerves and tissue some time to recover."

Aging arthritis patients find bone health crucial to their well-being. CBD has been proven to stimulate bone regeneration and to provide protection to other bones in the skeletal system. The *Journal of Bone Health* cited a study carried out by Dr. Yankel Gabet that showed that "CBD alone promotes 'markedly advanced' healing in broken bones by enhancing and speeding up the maturation of the collagenous matrix in the bone, a microstructure which provides the basis for mineralization of new bone tissue. With CBD therapy, according to Dr. Gabet's study, the broken bones will not only heal faster, but be harder to break than a bone left untreated with CBD."

Treating arthritis with CBD is a favorable step in the healing and treatment of rheumatoid arthritis and osteoarthritis. Since cannabinoids not only restores bone damage, but also manage pain and reduces tension, it is a desirable choice for suffering arthritics who want to find an alternative plan of treatment.

How to Use: According to the Mayo Clinic, the dosage recommended to treat chronic pain is 3 to 30 mg of CBD by mouth for an average of twenty-five days. Raw CBDA rich hemp extracts may also be effective. It is recommended to take anywhere from one to six servings (5 mg capsules or soft-gels) of CBDA daily. For treatment, resistant condition more concentrated gold hemp extract may also be needed. Hemp seed oil with omega 3 ALA in addition to marine omega 3 EPA and DHA may enhance benefits.

ATTENTION DEFICIT HYPERACTIVITY DISORDER

Attention deficit hyperactivity disorder (ADHD) is a common condition generally characterized by an inability to stay focused, pay attention, and control behavior. It is typically diagnosed in childhood but sometimes persists through adolescence and adulthood. ADHD affects about 11 percent of school-aged children and 2 to 5 percent of adults in the United States today.

It is important to note that in 1994, attention deficit disorder (ADD) was changed to "attention-deficit hyperactivity disorder," regardless of whether the individual showed symptoms of hyperactivity or not. The three types of ADHD are now identified as "predominately hyperactive-impulsive," "predominately inattentive," and "combined." A great many professionals and laypeople alike still use both terms, ADD and ADHD, interchangeably.

Symptoms
ADHD manifests itself differently in everyone. Other signs of the disorder may include:

- Excessive talking
- Fidgeting
- Forgetfulness
- Disorganization
- Hyperactivity

- Impulsivity
- Making careless mistakes

Triggers

Although there is no specific cause for these disorders, research has indicated that certain factors such as genetics, environment, and brain injury may play a role. In the majority of cases, children diagnosed with ADHD have a relative that has also been diagnosed with the condition. Exposure to toxic levels of lead have also been shown to contribute to ADHD.

Research has also suggested that there is a connection between nutrition and diet and ADHD symptoms. It is believed that food additives and sugar as well as a lack of omega-3 fatty acids may contribute to these symptoms.

Conventional Treatment/Side Effects

Generally, ADHD is treated with short-acting and long-acting stimulants, nonstimulants, and antidepressants. Stimulants, such as Ritalin, Adderall, and Dexedrine are the most common type of medication prescribed.

In the late 1990s, researchers discovered that methylphenidate, the active ingredient in Ritalin, treats ADHD symptoms by increasing dopamine levels in the brain. However, it was also discovered that Ritalin had a significant potential to cause permanent brain damage and psychiatric problems. Even non-stimulant ADHD drugs have serious psychiatric problems.

Although these stimulants may be effective in controlling and reducing the symptoms, as mentioned above there are some harmful side effects. Signs that may indicate problems are:

- Decreased appetite
- Delayed growth
- Headaches
- Irritability
- Moodiness
- Sleep problems
- Stomach Aches

CBD and Hemp Oil

Medical studies have demonstrated CBD's ability to reduce cortisol levels in the brain, which naturally causes an increase in dopamine levels. THC does this as well, but in a psychoactive way.

The results in treating ADHD with cannabis are often very significant. Research cites grades going from Cs and Ds to As and Bs. In almost all cases ADHD patients who were treated with cannabis gave an account of how it helped them pay attention, focus their attention, and stay on task. Dr. Bearman, a "figurehead of cannabis research," examined the relationship between the cannabinoid system and ADHD. His studies influenced the findings of the prospective therapeutic value of cannabinoids, which improve the brain's dopamine management systems.

How to Use: For a number of reasons, it is important to start slow and go slow. Starting with small amounts allows you more control in finding the optimum dose.

Administer CBD 2 hours apart from pharmaceuticals to help avert adverse medication interactions. To aid in its absorption, it should be taken with a high fat snack. Oils can be taken by syringe, in capsules, and through G-tubes. Less is often more with these situations and large amounts of CBD can cause anxiety in some cases. Look for a 100-mg spray product or drop that can deliver CBD per milligram. Some doctors have reported benefit with only a few sprays or 1 to 3 mg of CBD. THC would rarely be appropriate for this condition and almost never for a child. Hemp seed oil with omega 3 ALA in addition to marine omega 3 EPA and DHA may enhance benefits.

BLOOD CLOTS

Blood clots are clumps of blood that form as a result of an injury or cut, most commonly in the limbs. They can also form inside veins and arteries. If the clots break off they may become embedded in the heart, lungs, or brain. Clots forming inside your arteries may prevent oxygen from getting to your heart, lungs, or brain, resulting in life-threatening conditions.

Symptoms

Blood clots give differing symptoms depending on where in the body they appear. Many times blood clots will exist without any symptoms.

Leg or Arm

- Change in color
- Pain
- Swelling
- Tenderness
- Warm sensation

Heart

- Lightheadedness
- Severe pain in chest and/or arm
- Shortness of breath
- Sweating

Lungs

- Chest pain
- Coughing up blood
- Feeling dizzy
- Heart palpitations

- Problems breathing
- Shortness of breath
- Sweating

Brain

- Difficulty seeing
- Difficulty speaking

- Sudden, severe headache

Abdomen

- Bloody stools
- Diarrhea
- Nausea

- Severe pain and selling
- Vomiting

Triggers

Decrease in blood flow caused by clots may result in significant health problems. There are a number of risk factors and conditions that result from the formation of blood clots.

- Cancer and cancer treatments
- Dehydration
- Family history
- Immobility, prolonged
- Irregular heartbeat
- Medications
- Obesity

- Oral contraception
- Pregnancy
- Smoking
- Stroke
- Surgery
- Varicose veins

Conventional Treatment/Side Effects

Most commonly, blot clots are treated with anticoagulants or blood thinners. They prevent the clots from progressing and slow down the stretch of time it takes for blood to clot. The blood thinner most frequently prescribed is UF Heparin.

Although anticoagulants prevent new clots from forming and existing clots from growing, they may result in complications, such as internal bleeding, bruising, skin irritation at the sight of injection, bluish colored skin, and itching of the feet. If used over a long period of time, anticoagulants may cause osteoporosis.

CBD and Hemp Oil

Hemp oil is a natural blood thinner due to its omega-3 properties, helping to shorten and prevent blood clots. According to *Medical Marijuana Research,* "hemp could increase the anticoagulant effect of blood thinners by inhibiting its metabolism. It directly affects the anticoagulant properties of platelets in the blood. Therefore it naturally acts as a blood thinner and should rather be a replacement for blood thinning meds."

How to Use: If you are on blood thinners and would like to switch to hemp extracts, it is advisable to do so under the supervision of a physician. It is also important to take note that extracts with 2:1 THC to CBD ratio have been reported to be effective. Recommended dosage is between 3 mg to 30 mg of CBD taken daily.

See also: **HEADACHES; HEART DISEASE.**

CANCER

There are over a hundred different types of cancer. Cancer occurs when the cells in a body region begin dividing and spreading into surrounding tissues. It can appear anywhere inside the body. Many cancers form solid masses of tissue called *tumors*. There are two types of tumors: benign and malignant. Cancerous tumors are malignant and can invade or spread to nearby tissue. Benign tumors do not spread or invade nearby tissue, but they can be fairly large and depending upon their location, they can be life-threatening.

Symptoms

At the early stages of the cancer there may not be any noticeable signs or symptoms; however, as the disease develops, symptoms or signs may appear depending upon the cancer type, the stage, and the location. Common symptoms may include:

- Change in bowel habits
- Change in urination
- Fatigue
- Fever

- Loss of appetite
- Nausea
- Pain
- Persistent cough

- Skin changes
- Unexplained anemia
- Unusual lumps or discharge
- Vomiting
- Unexpected weight loss or weight gain

Triggers

Most cancers are due to environmental factors, while about 5 to 10 percent are due to genetic factors. This abnormal cell growth may be caused by the following:

- Autoimmune diseases
- Chemicals (carcinogens)
- Chronic inflammation
- Diet
- Genetics
- Hormones
- Infection
- Physical inactivity
- Radiation

Conventional Treatment/Side Effects

There are a number of conventional treatments for cancer. The kind of treatment prescribed will depend on the type of cancer and how advanced it is. These treatments include:

- Hormone therapy
- Immunotherapy
- Precision medicine
- Radiation therapy
- Stem cell transplant
- Surgery
- Targeted therapy

There are problems or side effects that appear when conventional cancer treatments affect healthy tissues or organs. Common side effects caused by cancer treatment may include:

- Anemia
- Appetite loss
- Bladder problems
- Bleeding (low platelets)
- Bruising easily
- Constipation
- Delirium
- Diarrhea
- Edema (water retention)
- Fatigue
- Hair Loss (Alopecia)
- Low white blood cells
- Lymphedema
- Mouth and throat problems
- Nerve problems (Peripheral Neuropathy)

- Pain
- Problem concentrating
- Sexual and fertility problems
- Skin and nail changes

- Sleep problems
- Urinary problems
- Vomiting

CBD and Hemp Oil

Cannabinoids offer patients a healing alternative in the treatment of extremely invasive cancers. Over twenty major research studies show that cannabinoids have anti-cancer properties with the potential to stop the growth of several different types of cancers, including melanoma, brain cancer, and breast cancer. Cannabinoids may also offset chemical toxicity from drugs and environmental sources, helping to preserve normal cells. Researchers at the University of Milan found that cannabidiol inhibits the growth of glioma cells, a type of brain tumor, in a dose-dependent manner, selectively targeting and killing malignant cells.

The medical establishment has also recognized the benefits of CBD for the side effects of chemotherapy. Studies have found that THC may also be advisable if the patient can tolerate it. Seek the guidance of a qualified health care provider with a proven track record and understanding of cannabinoids and cancer. Self-medication is ill advised and is not recommended. Hemp seed oil with omega 3 ALA in addition to marine omega 3 EPA and DHA may enhance benefits.

CARDIOVASCULAR DISEASE

See **HEART DISEASE.**

CHEMOTHERAPY, SIDE EFFECTS

See **CANCER.**

COLITIS, ULCERATIVE

See **ULCERATIVE COLITIS.**

CROHN'S DISEASE

Crohn's disease is a chronic, recurring inflammatory bowel disease (IBD) that primarily affects the lining of the gastrointestinal (GI) tract. Since the disease involves the immune system you may experience joint pain, eye problems, a skin rash, or liver disease. Crohn's can be painful and debilitating. With treatment, however, Crohn's patients can keep the disease in check.

Symptoms

Crohn's may be characterized by the following symptoms and signs ranging from mild to severe:

- Abdominal pain
- Anal fissures, Anemia, Bloody stools
- Diarrhea
- Fever, Malnutrition
- Nausea
- Obstruction in the bowel
- Weight loss

Triggers

The exact cause of Crohn's disease is unknown. Possible factors leading to the development of the disease have been connected to a combination of several elements, including problems with the immune system, genetics, and the environment.

Conventional Treatment/Side Effects

There is no cure for Crohn's disease. Medications are prescribed to control or prevent inflammation, and the choice of medication depends on the severity of the disease and whether complications exist.

Anti-inflammatory drugs are usually prescribed first, such as oral 5-aminosalicylates and corticosteroids (prednisone). Some side effects associated with anti-inflammatory drugs are upset stomach, nausea, vomiting, headache, dizziness, loss of appetite, and/or fatigue.

Immune system suppressors, such as Stelera, Tysabri, and Rheumatrex, also reduce inflammation. However, they should not be used long-term because of side effects, such as bloating, excessive facial hair, sleep disruption, and heightened risk of developing diabetes and osteoporosis.

When an infection is a consideration, antibiotics are prescribed, but there is no strong proof that they are effective for treating Crohn's disease. Common side effects experienced when taking an antibiotic include diarrhea, upset stomach, and nausea.

CBD and Hemp Oil

Cannabinoids have been found to lessen inflammation in the bowel, eventually reducing pain, providing nausea relief, and reducing feelings of unpleasantness. Present-day discoveries indicate that cannabinoid treatments are a significant competitor in the therapy and remission of Crohn's disease. In a 2005 pilot study, Tod Mikuriya, MD, and David Bearman, MD, questioned twelve Crohn's patients taking cannabis about their post-treatment symptoms. The patients reported a vast improvement in overall symptoms without adverse side effects.

How to Use: Recommended dosage is 3 to 30 mg daily. The reduction of stress and anxiety are critical for sufferers of inflammatory bowel disease.

DEPRESSION

We have all felt sad or down at one time or another, but sadness becomes problematic when it persists and negatively affects our life. Depression is one of the most common mental disorders. It is a mood disorder that affects almost all aspects of daily life. It may impact how you think, how you feel, and daily activities, such as sleeping, eating, and working.

Symptoms

According to the American Psychiatric Association, depression is characterized by "a deep feeling of sadness or a marked loss of interest or pleasure in activities." Common symptoms that usually are associated with depression may include:

- Feelings of hopelessness and worthlessness
- Loss of interest in social activities and daily activities
- Change in appetite
- Restlessness and irritability
- Chronic fatigue
- Feeling lethargic
- Unexplained aches and pains
- Unexplained crying and anger outbursts
- Lack of appetite or eating too much
- Inability to focus
- Excessive sleep or insomnia
- Thoughts of suicide
- Moodiness
- Loss of interest in sex

Triggers

Research has made clear that depression is a serious illness caused by changes in brain chemistry. Many factors can contribute to the onset of depression, including genetics, changes in hormone levels, certain medical conditions, stress, grief, difficult life circumstances, or substance abuse. The depression may be triggered by one or a combination of factors.

Conventional Treatment/Side Effects

Traditionally, treatment for depression includes forms of psychotherapy and/or medications. There are a number of forms of psychotherapy that are used, such as cognitive-behavioral therapy (CBT), which works to replace negative thought patterns with more grounded and useful ones.

The most common medications prescribed are called selective serotonin re-uptake inhibitors (SSRIs). Prozac (fluoxetine), Paxil (paroxetine), Zoloft (sertraline) and Luvox (fluvoxamine) are the most popular brands. Although SSRI antidepressant medications seem to be safe, many people will experience side effects while taking them, such as nausea, diarrhea, agitation, insomnia, headache, or decreased sex drive. Long-term side effects of taking SSRI medications may include difficulties sleeping, sexual dysfunction, and weight gain.

CBD and Hemp Oil

The endocannabinoid system in our brain helps to balance mood and influence our "reward-seeking behavior." It also helps maintain balance in the body by reducing stress and regulating sleep and appetite. Depression can negatively impact the endocannabinoid system, resulting in poor sleep and eating habits, as well as high levels of stress. Researchers at the University of Buffalo have found that using cannabidiol to restore endocannabinoid function may help to stabilize mood and treat depression. Cannabis use has been proven to ease stress, help insomnia, and regulate appetite.

Although anyone can use CBD to manage depression, it is advisable to consult your doctor or medical caregiver if you are pregnant or suffering from other diseases. If you are considering changing from traditional pharmaceuticals to hemp oil or CBD, it is also important to solicit advice from your physician or medical caregiver.

How to Use: Recommended dosage is 3 to 45 mg. Raw CBDA may also add support. Hemp seed oil with omega 3 ALA in addition to marine omega 3 EPA and DHA may enhance benefits. Additional Omega 3 EPA would be recommended.

DERMATITIS, ATOPIC

See ECZMA. Cytokines (proteins), INF-gamma and TNF-alpha, and significantly reduced the severity of insulitis (see below) compared to non-treated controls.

Use 3 to 30 mg CBD until symptoms are relieved. Be sure to decrease the amount of CBD with any worsening of symptoms. Hemp seed oil with omega 3 ALA in addition to marine omega 3 EPA and DHA may enhance benefits.

ECZEMA

Atopic dermatitis (eczema) is a skin condition that makes your skin red and itchy. It is common in children but can occur at any age. Eczema is chronic and tends to flare periodically and then subside.

Eczema affects about 10 to 20 percent of infants and about 3 percent of adults and children in the United States. No cure has been found for the condition.

Symptoms

Eczema most often begins before the age of five and may persist into adolescence and adulthood. For some people, it flares periodically and then clears up for a time, even for several years. The following are symptoms that are associated with eczema and the damage it can cause:

- Itching, especially at night
- Raw, sensitive, swollen skin from scratching
- Red to brownish-gray patches
- Small, raised bumps, which may leak fluid and crust over when scratched
- Thickened, cracked, dry, scaly skin

Triggers

Factors that can worsen eczema signs and symptoms include:

- Bacteria and viruses
- Dry skin from long, hot baths and showers
- Dust and pollen
- Eggs, milk, peanuts, soybeans, fish, and wheat, in infants and children
- Heat and humidity changes
- Solvents, cleaners, soaps, and detergent

- Stress
- Sweating

- Tobacco smoke and air pollution
- Wool clothing, blankets, and carpets

Conventional Treatment/Side Effects

Since a cure for eczema has not yet been found, the first line of approach by most general practitioners and dermatologists is to prescribe topical corticosteroids. These are steroids that are applied in a cream or gel base to the areas of eczema on the skin. Some people have an allergic response to the steroids themselves, which can result in itching, white bumps, and a rash that resembles acne. Eczema can also become tolerant to steroids and reappear despite continued application.

Some of the following side effects can also be associated with the use of corticosteroid cream:

- Impaired wound healing
- Secondary infection

- Skin thinning

In addition to the use of corticosteroids, other conventional methods of treating eczema include: topical calcineurin inhibitors, as well as antibiotics, antifungals, anti-histamines, antivirals, and emollients. However, no conventional treatments offer permanent resolutions and have far more limitations and side effects than alternative methods and treatments.

CBD and Hemp Oil

Hemp seed oil is rich in essential fatty acids omega-6 and omega-3, which help maintain good skin health by keeping cell membranes flexible.

In 2005, the *Journal of Dermatology Treatment* published a study done by Dr. J. Callaway on the treatment of eczema. Dr. Callaway found that the symptoms of skin dryness and itching significantly improved in patients suffering from eczema after using hemp seed oil for 20 weeks. He stated, "We saw remarkable reduction in dryness, itching, and an overall improvement in symptoms."

How to Use: Dr. Callaway discovered that 2 tablespoons of dietary hemp seed oil consumed daily can help relieve the effects of eczema. As the dosage of CBD differs for each person, it is best to start small and gradually increase until you experience the desired result. CBDA rich topical balms are reported to be effective in the treatment of eczema. Topical gold concentrates may also be required for treatment resistant cases. Isolated CBD crystals may produce topical products that are more drug like and corrective than natural daily use products. 3 to 15 mg of CBD twice daily for internal inflammation. Hemp seed oil with omega 3 ALA in addition to marine omega 3 EPA and DHA may enhance benefits.

EPILEPSY

Epilepsy is a chronic neurological disorder that is characterized by recurrent, unprovoked episodes of convulsions, known as seizures, or loss of consciousness. It can affect people of all ages. There are many types of seizures, which are typically classified by physicians as either generalized, focal, or unknown. Seizures usually last from a few seconds to a few minutes.

Symptoms

Seizures usually occur without warning. The symptoms may vary depending on the type. Usually, someone suffering from seizures will experience the same kind of seizure each time. Therefore, the symptoms will appear similar for each episode. The signs and symptoms may include:

- Changes in sensations (waves of heat or cold)
- Dazed behavior
- Heart racing
- Loss of awareness
- Loss of consciousness
- Muscles jerk out of control or twitch (arms and legs)
- Temporary confusion
- Weakening of muscles

Triggers

What causes the disorder may differ by the age of the person. If no clear cause is apparent, it may be a genetic factor. Common triggers of epileptic seizures may include:

Infants and Children

- Born with brain malformations
- Congenital disorders
- Drug use by mother
- Fever
- Head trauma
- Infections
- Intracranial hemorrhage
- Lack of oxygen during birth

Adults

- Alzheimer's disease
- Head injuries

- Stroke   - Tumors

- Trauma

Conventional Treatment/Side Effects

A large number of epileptic seizures are controlled by anticonvulsant drugs. The choice of anticonvulsant drug prescribed will depend on the person's age, overall health, and medical history. Although the drugs can control the seizures, they don't cure the disorder and most often people will need to continue taking the medication. Use of the drugs may result in adverse side effects such as dizziness, fatigue, nausea, vomiting, rash, depression, and loss of appetite.

CBD and Hemp Oil

Evidence from studies demonstrate that CBD could potentially be helpful in controlling seizures. The research has shown that CBD can act as an anticonvulsant and may even have antipsychotic effects. A number of studies have shown the use of CBD to be an effective method of reducing the number of seizures a person with epilepsy experiences.

One such study is that of Dr. Anup Patel, of Nationwide Children's Hospital and The Ohio State University College of Medicine in Columbus, who found that cannabidiol is an effective treatment for Lennox-Gastaut syndrome, a serious form of epilepsy. A group of 225 young patients with Lennox-Gastaut syndrome were tested. Each day, patients were administered either a higher or lower dose of cannabidiol, or an inactive placebo. The patients who took the higher dose experienced a 42 percent reduction in drop seizures overall. Furthermore, 40 percent of patients in that group saw that the amount of seizures they usually experienced was reduced by half or more. The patients who took the lower dose had a 37 percent reduction in drop seizures overall, with 36 percent experiencing less than half the usual amount of seizures. In contrast, those in the placebo group had a 17 percent reduction in drop seizures overall, with 15 percent seeing that their seizures were reduced by half or more.

More research needs to be completed to study the safety and efficacy of CBD, however the medical community is beginning to recognize the positive outcomes that some people have experienced from CBD rich extracts.

How to Use: Recommended dose is 30 mg. Self-medication is ill advised especially when taking multiple anti-epileptic medications. The drug-to-drug interactions with CBD in this patient population requires very strict medical monitoring, supervision and care. Reports of miraculous cures are followed up years later to reveal another wall of treatment resistance has been hit and that the miracle cannabis strain no longer works. Hearts are broken, the promise of hemp is no longer kept, it fails to deliver. What suddenly changed? Our ECS, that's what changed, especially when we are very sick. The ECS may be our master control system, yet we never learn how to fully control it and may even do harm while attempting to heal.

FDA-approved CBD drugs are being developed for treatment resistant seizures that have no commercial counterpart or generics in the market today. These FDA-approved CBD drugs are not hemp extracts and will only be available at pharmacies. When treating epilepsy with CBD, the only product to ever be used must be filled at a pharmacy with a childproof cap. It is not recommended to use hemp extracts sold on line or independent natural retailers.

EYE DISORDERS

See **AGE-RELATED MACULAR DEGENERATION; GLAUCOMA.**

FIBROMYALGIA

Fibromyalgia (FM) is a common condition that is characterized by chronic pain and tenderness in the muscles and bones, as well as fatigue. It mostly affects women, although men and children can also suffer from the condition. It can be a difficult disorder to diagnose because the main symptoms may be similar to symptoms of other conditions.

Symptoms

Pain is the main symptom and felt at different degrees at different times of the day. For some the pain is at its worse when they awake and improves as the day progresses. Different people may experience this pain in various ways, such as chronic, all-over, shooting, tender, aching and deep pain.

Other common symptoms associated with FM may be:

- Anxiety
- Chronic fatigue
- Cognitive problems ("fibro fog")
- Depression
- Irritable bowel symptoms
- Migraines
- Restless leg
- Trouble sleeping

Triggers

Doctors aren't able to find a direct link related to FM, however a combination of factors may play a role in triggering the condition, including:

- Emotional trauma

- Family history

- Genetics

- Infections

- Physical trauma

- Sex (diagnosed more often in women)

Conventional Treatment/Side Effects

Commonly a healthcare provider will recommend medication or therapy to help reduce the symptoms associated with fibromyalgia. The common choices of medication are over-the-counter pain relievers, such as acetaminophen, ibuprofen, or naproxen sodium and antidepressants, such as Cymbalta. A prescription drug, such as tramadol, may also be recommended for pain relief.

Besides medications, a number of therapies (traditional and alternative) may be suggested to decrease the effects of the condition on your body, including physical therapy, occupational therapy, acupuncture, yoga, or tai chi.

Over-the-counter medications, like all drugs, can cause side effects and may not be safe for everyone. The side effects generally include stomach upset or pain, nausea, diarrhea, or heartburn. In some cases, it may raise blood pressure, result in stomach ulcers or bleeding, or cause allergic reactions.

CBD and Hemp Oil

Although there is a lack of scientific research, some recent reports have shown that people suffering from fibromyalgia have managed a number of symptoms with CBD oil. These reports cite that these patients were able to find relief from chronic pain, anxiety, depression, mood swings, and difficulty sleeping without the side effects of traditional drugs.

How to Use: As recommended by the CBD Oil Review, to treat chronic pain take 3 to 30 mg CBD by mouth for an average of 25 days. As serving size or dosage of CBD differs for each person, it is suggested to start small and gradually increase until you experience the desired result. Topical balms may also offer relief from pain, inflammation, and swelling. Hemp seed oil with omega 3 ALA in addition to marine omega 3 EPA and DHA may enhance benefits.

FM

See **FIBROMYALGIA.**

GLAUCOMA

Glaucoma is indicated when there has been damage to the optic nerve of the eye. It is the leading cause of blindness in people over the age of 60 years old. There are two types of glaucoma: primary open-angle, which is the most common, and closed-angle or narrow-angle.

Symptoms

In the early stages of open-angle glaucoma, there aren't any obvious signs or symptoms. On the other hand, symptoms for an attack of closed-angle glaucoma may include:

- Appearance of rainbows or halos
- Decreased vision
- Eye pain or pain in forehead
- Eye redness
- Hazy or blurred vision
- Headache
- Nausea
- Vomiting
- Tunnel vision

Triggers

Glaucoma occurs when fluid builds up in the front part of your eye. That extra fluid increases the pressure in your eye, damaging the optic nerve and causing vision loss. The reason for the buildup may include:

- Blocked blood vessels in the eye
- Eye infections (severe)
- Genetics
- Inflammation
- Injury to the eye, blunt or chemical

Conventional Treatment/Side Effects

Glaucoma is most commonly treated with eye drops. Although these eye drops decrease pressure by helping the fluid drain, they may cause some side effects, such as stinging or itching, dry mouth, blurred vision, and changes in energy level, heartbeat, and pulse.

An oral medication, usually a carbonic anhydrase inhibitor, may be prescribed as well if the eye drops don't decrease the pressure. Side effects include depression, upset stomach, kidney stones, frequent urination, and a tingling sensation in the toes and fingers. If the oral medication or eye drops fail to improve the patient's condition, surgery (laser or traditional) may be necessary.

CBD and Hemp Oil

Animal studies have shown that CBD has been proven to be beneficial in decreasing intraocular pressure. One study, cited in *Graefe's Archive for Clinical and Experimental Ophthalmology* in 2000, stated that "applied cannabinoids directly to the eyes of rabbits recorded decreased intraocular pressure within 1.5 hours of administration and the effects lasted for more than 6 hours. In addition, the eye to which the cannabinoid had not been administered also experienced a decrease in intraocular pressure, but the effect lasted for 4 hours."

Scientific research submitted to the *European Journal of Neuroscience* found that "applying a cannabinoid directly to the human eye decreased intraocular pressure within 30 minutes and reached maximal reduction in the first 60 minutes." These studies, as well as other observations conducted, confirm that cannabinoids may decrease the intraocular pressure in the eye when administered topically or systemically.

How to Use: The recommended treatment for glaucoma is a single CBD dose of 15 to 30 mg. THC may be required. Hemp seed oil with omega 3 ALA in addition to marine omega 3 EPA and DHA may enhance benefits.

HEADACHE

Many people experience headaches at some point in their life. They can range from mild to very severe and can negatively impact anyone. The severity and the location of the pain are associated with the type of headache, such as tension headaches, cluster headaches, sinus headaches, rebound headaches, and migraine headaches.

Symptoms

The following signs or symptoms are characteristic of each kind of headache:

- **Cluster headache:** (occurs in groups) severe pain on one side of head, watery eye and nasal congestion or runny nose on that same side

- **Migraine headaches:** one sided, throbbing pain with a sensitivity to light and that may be accompanied by nausea and/or vomiting

- **Rebound headaches:** dull, tension-type headache or a more severe migraine-like headache

- **Sinus headache:** pain and pressure in sinuses and may be accompanied by fever

- **Tension headache** (most common): mild, moderate, or intense pain or pressure around the temples or back of head or neck

Triggers

Headaches are primarily caused by an inflammation of the blood vessels in and around the brain and/or the chemical activity in your brain. Triggers may be lifestyle factors and/ or a concealed disease, including:

- Alcohol
- Too much caffeine
- Changes in waking/sleeping patterns
- Dehydration
- Food additives
- Hormonal changes in women
- Infections
- Lack of exercise
- Medication overuse (rebound headache)
- Personality traits
- Skipping meals
- Sleep deprivation
- Stress

Conventional Treatment/Side Effects

Traditional headache treatment depends on the type of headache you're fighting. Tension headaches may be treated with over-the-counter pain killers, such as aspirin, ibuprofen and acetaminophen. The same over-the-counter medications may help to relieve pain from a migraine, although certain prescription medications also exist, such as Imitrex or Zomig. Cluster headaches usually require injectable prescribed medications (for example, Imitrex and Sumavel) or prescribed nasal sprays (Zomig or Imitrex) which provide quick relief. The over-the-counter pain killers or nasal decongestants may help relieve pain from sinus headaches.

Although you may experience relief from headache pain, these common drugs may trigger nausea, sleepiness, fatigue, or a racing heartbeat. Use of these medications over a long period of time may result in rebound headaches.

CBD and Hemp Oil

Hemp oil and other CBD products exhibit the ability to treat headaches and migraines. Studies have indicated a relationship between migraines and endocannabinoid dysfunction. In a survey conducted by SFGate, 100 percent of the population reported that CBD oil relieved their migraines.

At the University of Perugia in 2007, researchers found that the endocannabinoid levels in the cerebrospinal fluid of patients suffering from chronic migraines were quite low, inferring that an impairment of the endocannabinoid system might result in chronic headpain. Neurologist and cannabinoid researcher Dr. Ethan Russo took the relationship between endocannabinoid deficiency and migraines to develop the Clinical Endocannabinoid Theory. According to Dr. Russo's theory, plant-based cannabinoids like CBD can help restore balance to the endocannabinoid system.

How to Use: 15 mg to 30 mg of CBD twice daily is recommended. Vaping has also been reported to be an effective way to deliver fast relief with either CBD or THC, if the patient can tolerate THC. Hemp seed oil with omega 3 ALA in addition to marine omega 3 EPA and DHA may enhance benefits.

HEART DISEASE

Heart disease, or cardiovascular disease, is the leading cause of death in the United States and currently affects over 80 million Americans. It refers to any condition that affects the heart and blood vessels. Coronary artery disease, angina pectoris, atherosclerosis, congestive heart failure, and heart arrhythmias are among the most common cardiovascular conditions.

Symptoms

Symptoms of heart disease are generally caused by narrowed blood vessels or an abnormal heartbeat. People are often not aware that they have a heart condition until an emergency such as a heart attack or heart failure occurs. Common symptoms include:

- Bradycardia (slow heartbeat)
- Chest pain (angina)

- Dizziness
- Fainting

- Lightheadedness
- Pain in neck, jaw, throat, or back
- Pain or numbness in legs or arms

- Shortness of breath
- Tachycardia (racing heartbeat)

Triggers

Along with genetics, which is a significant contributor, other common factors that can cause heart disease include:

- Chronic stress
- Diabetes
- Excessive alcohol/drug use
- High blood pressure
- High cholesterol

- Obesity
- Physical inactivity
- Poor diet
- Smoking

Conventional Treatment/Side Effects

Diagnosis and treatment of various heart conditions will vary. Along with suggesting lifestyle changes, such as eating a healthy low-fat diet and incorporating a moderate exercise program, physicians may also recommend medication. Included among the most commonly prescribed conventional medications for heart disease are ACE inhibitors to widen arteries, vasodilators to allow easier blood flow through the vessels, and blood thinners to prevent the formation of clots.

The possible side effects of ACE inhibitors may include dizziness, fatigue, and rapid heartbeat. Common side effects associated with vasodilators are edema (fluid retention), heart palpitations, joint and chest pain, headaches, and nausea. Blood thinners increase the risk of bleeding, which can be life-threatening. Do not take blood thinners if you have a bleeding disorder like hemophilia, stomach or intestinal bleeding, an ulcer, or very high blood pressure. Avoid them if you have had recent or upcoming surgery or dental work; a recent head injury or aneurysm; or severe heart disease. Pregnant women should avoid blood thinners as they have been linked to birth defects. Many drugs can have serious interactions when taken with warfarin or heparin. Before taking any blood thinner, be sure to inform your doctor about any and all medications you are currently taking or have used recently. Any type of heart medication should always be taken under the watchful eye of a doctor or other health care professional.

CBD and Hemp Oil

CBD oil could prove to be very helpful in treating heart disease. Because of its anti-inflammatory properties, CBD can help relax the blood vessels, allowing blood to flow through more easily. It has shown positive effects in patients with ischemia, or an insufficient supply of blood to the heart muscles. CBD has proven effective in patients who have heart disease caused by diabetes and stroke. It reduces the cardiovascular response to stress and has a direct effect on the longevity of white blood cells.

A 2013 article issued in the *British Journal of Clinical Pharmacology* produced data that showed the positive role CBD plays in the treatment of heart disease. CBD is known to reduce tension on blood vessel walls. *In vivo* CBD treatments in the heart have been shown to reduce the amount of dead tissue created by lack of blood supply, known as infarct. As cited in a recent study published in the *Journal of Agricultural and Food Chemistry*, hemp oil contains a high concentration of sterols that may help reduce risk of heart disease and promote heart health.

How to Use: Recommended dosage is 3 to 30 mg of CBD taken daily. Check with your healthcare provider before taking CBD.

HIGH BLOOD PRESSURE

High blood pressure, or hypertension, affects nearly 30 percent of people in the U.S. alone. Involving the force of blood flow, hypertension can damage arteries and lead to life-threatening conditions like heart disease and stroke. A blood pressure reading is shown as two numbers—a top number, which shows the force of blood flow when the heart is beating (systolic pressure); and a lower number, which shows the force when the heart is resting (diastolic pressure). According to the current recommendations of the American Heart Association, a reading under 120/80 is considered normal, while a reading of 140/90 or above is considered high. One frightening aspect of hypertension is that it doesn't exhibit any obvious symptoms. Because of this, many people are unaware that they have it, which is why it is sometimes called "the silent killer." High blood pressure cannot be cured, but it can be managed successfully.

Symptoms

Typically, high blood pressure does not exhibit any unusual symptoms. The only way to know for certain if you have it is to have your physician take a reading. Some common inconclusive symptoms can include:

- Blood spots on the eyes
- Chest pains
- Facial flushing
- Fatigue

- Nosebleeds
- Severe headaches
- Shortness of breath

Triggers

Common factors that can cause high blood pressure include:

- Age (older people are more likely to develop high blood pressure)
- Genetics/family history
- Excessive alcohol use

- High sodium/low potassium diet
- Obesity
- Physical inactivity
- Smoking
- Stress

Conventional Treatment/Side Effects

To treat high blood pressure, doctors will often first suggest making some basic lifestyle changes, such as eating a healthy low-sodium diet and exercising regularly. Quitting smoking and reducing or eliminating alcohol use can also help to reduce high blood pressure. The most common recommended medications include diuretics, or water pills. Diuretics help reduce blood volume by eliminating excess sodium and water from the body. Beta blockers, which often work in combination with other drugs, are prescribed to help open blood vessels and reduce pressure on the heart. Angiotensin II receptor blockers (ARBs) and calcium channel blockers help relax blood vessels to allow easier blood flow.

Beta blockers may cause drowsiness, dizziness, dry mouth, and constipation or diarrhea. Fatigue, headaches, dizziness, and dry cough are common reactions to ARBs, while calcium channel blockers may cause lightheadedness, constipation, swelling of feet and ankles, and increased appetite. Grapefruit and grapefruit juice interacts negatively with calcium channel blockers and must be avoided. Alcohol should also be avoided as it interferes with the drug's positive effects while increasing its side effects.

CBD and Hemp Oil

Recent research suggests that the body's cannabinoid system plays a significant role in controlling blood pressure. Animal studies have demonstrated that endocannabinoids suppress hypertension and reduce blood pressure.

In a study originally published in 2015, Christopher Stanley and his team at the University of Nottingham School of Medicine set out to discover if endocannabinoids could be the future replacement for today's commonly used high blood pressure drugs. The aim of the study was to determine the effects of CBD on blood vessels. The results of this study brought further insight into CBD's impact on the body's internal endocannabinoid system: the endocannabinoid receptors proved to play a vital role blood vessel constriction and relaxation. In a constricted vessel, activation of CB1 receptors with CBD caused the vessels to relax and dilate, thus lowering blood pressure.

In an article cited in the *British Journal of Clinical Pharmacology* in 2012, evidence suggested that CBD is beneficial in the workings of the cardiovascular system. The animal study showed that CBD protects against the vascular damage caused by a high glucose environment, inflammation, and type 2 diabetes, as well as aids in the vascular permeability (the ability of a blood vessel wall to allow the flow of small molecules and whole cells) associated with such environments.

How to Use: Recommended dosage is 3 to 30 mg of CBD taken twice daily. If you are taking medication for blood pressure, you should consult your doctor before taking CBD.

INFLAMMATION

Inflammation is the immune system's attempt to heal the body after an injury, defend it against foreign invaders like viruses and bacteria, and repair damaged tissue. During this process, the body's white blood cells are released into the bloodstream and travel to the affected area, where they (along with hormones and nutrients) attack the harmful invaders and begin the healing process.

Inflammation can be acute or chronic, and can occur internally or externally. *Acute inflammation* is short-term and activated by such injuries as a cut on the skin, a sprained ankle, or a stubbed toe; as well as a bacterial or viral infection. The inflammatory process involves increased blood flow to the affected area, and often results in swelling, warmth, redness, and pain. *Chronic inflammation* is long-term. It can result from failure to eliminate the cause of an acute inflammation or it can be from a persistent, unresolved low-intensity irritant. Often, chronic inflammation is caused by a faulty autoimmune response that attacks healthy tissue, mistaking it as harmful.

Asthma, rheumatoid arthritis, and ulcerative colitis are just a few of the hundreds of autoimmune disorders, and nearly all include inflammation as one of the symptoms. Chronic inflammation has also been implicated as a contributor to such serious illnesses as heart disease, stroke, and certain cancers.

Symptoms

The acronym PRISH refers to the five most significant symptoms of acute inflammation: Pain, Redness, Immobility (loss of joint function), Swelling, and Heat. For chronic inflammation, the symptoms are not always as apparent. They usually occur when the associated disease or health condition presents itself. Some of the more common symptoms have included constant or ongoing:

- Depression
- Fatigue

- Joint or muscle pain
- Stomach/gastrointestinal pain

Triggers

Typically the symptom of a broader disease or condition (often in the gut), chronic inflammation may be triggered by:

- Allergies, food and environmental
- Autoimmune disorders
- Digestive issues
- Environmental toxins (heavy metals)

- Hormone imbalance
- Obesity
- Poor diet (processed, sugary, fast foods)
- Sleep deprivation
- Stress, emotional and physical

Conventional Treatment/Side Effects

Symptoms of acute inflammation are often treated with over-the-counter nonsteroidal anti-inflammatory drugs (NSAIDs), such as aspirin and ibuprofen. These drugs, however, are associated with a number of possible side effects, including dizziness, stomach pain, ringing in the ears, high blood pressure, and the onset of stomach ulcers.

Corticosteroids such as prednisone may be prescribed to treat a number of inflammatory diseases and conditions. Taken orally, by injection, or applied topically, corticosteroids can be effective, but they also carry the risk of serious side effects. High blood pressure, edema (fluid retention), osteoporosis, cataracts, weight gain, and memory issues are among the most common.

CBD and Hemp Oil

Ongoing research indicates that hemp and CBD oils may be effective in treating inflammatory conditions—without the serious side effects and health complications affiliated with conventional treatments. Hemp oil's high content of omega-3 fatty acids is one of the reasons for this effectiveness. Omega-3s slow down and block the enzymes that produce prostaglandins, which cause inflammation.

A 2006 study that appeared in the *European Journal of Pharmacology* set out to determine the effect of cannabidiol as an effective treatment in managing chronic inflammatory and neuropathic (nerve) pain in laboratory rats. After pain was induced in the study subjects, they were given oral doses of CBD. After seven days of repeated treatment, the subjects showed a reduction in pain and inflammation. The results indicated that CBD may indirectly affect the cannabinoid receptors in the brain—CB1 and CB2—that help to manage pain.

Results of a study done at the University of Mississippi Medical Center and published in the *Free Radical Biology & Medicine Journal* showed that cannabidiol can be helpful in reducing the impact of inflammation on oxidative stress. Oxidative stress and inflammation are known contributors to a number of conditions, including high blood pressure, rheumatoid arthritis, Type 1 and Type 2 diabetes, atherosclerosis, depression, and Alzheimer's disease.

How to Use: Recommended dosage is 3 to 45 mg. Combine CBDA and CBD with THC for those who can tolerate THC. Never self-medicate with THC. Make sure you are guided by a qualified physician. Topical balms and concentrates may be effective for inflammatory conditions of the skin. Hemp seed oil with omega 3 ALA in addition to marine omega 3 EPA and DHA may enhance benefits.

Depending on the dosage and the person, CBD can be stimulating if taken prior to sleep, while some people report dramatic improvements in sleep quality. The best way to determine if hemp extracts will help you fall and stay asleep is to slowly titrate with drops or sprays, gradually increasing the dose to achieve the desired effect. Some people find it more beneficial to start the day with CBD due to its effects on the neurotransmitter serotonin, while other report best results one hour prior to bed time. Hemp seed oil with omega 3 ALA in addition to marine omega 3 EPA and DHA may enhance benefits.

IRRITABLE BOWEL SYNDROME

An estimated 35 million Americans suffer from irritable bowel syndrome (IBS)—a chronic gastrointestinal condition in which the intestines do not function properly. Normally, waste moves through the intestines and is eliminated from the body thanks to the rhythmic muscular contractions of the intestines. With IBS, the contractions are irregular and erratic—either too strong or not strong enough. This results in a number of uncomfortable, often severe symptoms that typically include abdominal pain, cramping, bloating, and diarrhea and/or constipation. In many cases, the gastrointestinal tract is sensitive to certain dietary influences, which further complicates the condition. Unlike Crohn's disease and ulcerative colitis, which are serious inflammatory bowel diseases, IBS is considered a functional problem of the intestines.

There is no specific test for diagnosing IBS. The condition is generally diagnosed by eliminating more serious problems, such as diverticulitis, ulcerative colitis, and colorectal cancer, which can produce symptoms that are similar to IBS. Its diagnosis is also based on the duration and frequency of the symptoms, which occur at least three times a month for at least six months.

Symptoms

The signs and symptoms of IBS, as well as their severity, will vary. Typically they occur after eating, and include:

- Abdominal pain
- Bloating
- Cramping
- Diarrhea and/or constipation
- Gas
- Loss of appetite
- Mucus in the stool
- Nausea
- Painful bowel movements

Triggers

Although the cause of this condition is unknown, the following factors have been known to trigger or worsen the attacks:

- Anxiety
- Artificial sweeteners
- Caffeinated, carbonated, and alcoholic beverages
- Food sensitivities (often gluten)
- Lactose intolerance
- Overgrowth of intestinal bacteria
- Stress

Conventional Treatment/Side Effects

Dietary modifications are typically the first recommendation for those with IBS. Avoiding trigger foods and maintaining a high-fiber diet based on vegetables and whole grains can help reduce or prevent an IBS flare up. If the problem persists, medication may be suggested. The doctor may recommend an anti-diarrheal like loperimide (Imodium), which slows the movement of the digestive tract, allowing more time for the reabsorption of water from the stool. This type of medication does not reduce the pain or bloating associated with the diarrhea, and it can cause dizziness, dry mouth, and fatigue. In some people, it can initiate severe constipation, nausea, and irregular heartbeat. To help prevent bowel spasms, medications such as dicyclomine (Bentyl) and hyoscyamine (Levsin) may be prescribed; however, they must be taken with caution as they can make urinating difficult and worsen constipation. For those with constipation, a laxative may help treat the symptoms, but not necessarily the pain.

CBD and Hemp Oil

In addition to producing a calming effect in patients, CBD works as a powerful anti-spasmodic, which helps relieve the pain associated with irritable bowel syndrome. Recent research has shown that cannabinoids play a crucial role in controlling gastrointestinal inflammation and motility. According to an abstract that appeared in *European Review for Medical and Pharmacological Sciences*, "Consistently, in vivo studies have shown that cannabinoids reduce gastrointestinal transit in rodents through activation of CB1 receptors. . . . Cannabinoids also reduce gastrointestinal motility in randomized clinical trials."

Many people with IBS suffer from anxiety and depression. While the psychoactive THC component of the cannabis plant has been shown to raise mental spirits, a 2016 study showed the same results with CBD—the plant's non psychoactive component. Minutes after the study's rodent subjects were given a single dose of CBD, they displayed signs of reduced anti-social and anxiety-like behavior.

An article in the May 2013 issue of *Phytotherapy Research* cited CBD as "a promising drug for the therapy of inflammatory bowel diseases." CBD is continuously touted for its anti-inflammatory properties and shows great potential as a treatment for IBD and other gut disturbances.

How to Use: 10 to 15 mg of CBD taken daily. 15 mg gold soft-gels have also been reported to be effective. THC may be helpful if the patient can tolerate it and is under a physician's care. Excessive oils may not be tolerated, so look for ultra-high omega 3 EPA and DHA to support the ECS and the inflammatory response.

MACULAR DEGENERATION

See **AGE-RELATED MACULAR DEGENERATION.**

MENOPAUSE

See **HORMONAL IMBALANCE.**

MIGRAINE HEADACHE

See **HEADACHE.**

MS

See **MULTIPLE SCLEROSIS.**

MULTIPLE SCLEROSIS

Multiple sclerosis (MS) is a disease of the central nervous system in which the immune system attacks nerve fibers in the body. The breakdown of the protective nerve fiber sheath causes miscommunications between your brain and the rest of your body, damages nerves, and can potentially disable the spinal cord.

Symptoms

The symptoms of MS depend on how badly the nerves are damaged. Severe MS can cause a patient to lose the ability to walk, while patients with mild MS may only experience numbness. The most common symptoms, both mild and severe, are listed below:

- Bowel and bladder function problems
- Dizziness
- Fatigue
- Numbness or weakness (often occurring on one side of the body at a time)

- Paralysis
- Partial or complete vision loss
- Shock-like sensations in the neck

- Slurred speech
- Tremor and a lack of coordination

Triggers

It is not known what causes MS, although it is classified as an autoimmune disease. Some of the possible risk factors are the following:

- Age (onset is typically between the ages of 15 and 60)
- Climate and environment (MS is more common in temperate-climate areas)
- Gender (women are twice as likely as men to develop MS)
- Genetics/family history
- Having certain autoimmune diseases
- Having certain infections, such as Epstein-Barr virus
- Race (white people have the highest rates of MS)

Conventional Treatment/Side Effects

Currently there are no effective medications or treatments for MS. Treatments are mainly given to ease the painful symptoms and make patients more comfortable, or to slow down the disease's progression. Such treatments include corticosteroids, taken orally or through an IV, which reduce inflammation in the nerves. Another treatment is plasma exchange, in which the plasma in your blood is separated from the blood cells. The blood cells are mixed with albumin, a protein solution, and then filtered back into your body.

Treatments to slow MS's progression include ocrelizumab, which is the only FDA-approved therapy for primary-progressive MS. Having primary-progressive MS means that the disease worsens from the onset, without relapses or remissions. Ocrelizumab is an antibody medication and has been shown in trials to impede the disability from becoming worse.

Patients with relapsing-remitting MS, meanwhile, experience intermittent attacks of neurological symptoms followed by periods of remission. Ocrelizumab can also be used to treat this form of MS because it has been shown to reduce the amount of relapses someone experiences. Other treatments for this form of MS are beta interferons, which are injections that can reduce the severity of relapses; glatiramer acetate, which is also injected and has been shown to block the immune system from attacking the nerve fibers; and dimethyl fumarate, which is an oral medication that may reduce relapses.

Other therapies for MS include physical therapy to strengthen the weakened muscles and improve mobility; muscle relaxants; and anti-fatigue medications. The American Academy of Neurology recommends oral cannabis extract to treat symptoms of muscle spasticity and pain. Below, we will look more into the literature surrounding CBD's use in treating MS.

CBD and Hemp Oil

Dozens of studies have been published illustrating the benefits of CBD on the symptoms of MS. Much of the research has been performed using Sativex, a medication that consists of THC and CBD in a 1:1 ratio. Sativex may become the first FDA-approved prescription marijuana extract.

In 2011, a drug profile for Sativex was published in the *Expert Review of Neurotherapeutics.* In the profile, the authors detailed what Sativex is (a 1:1 mix of THC and CBD available as an oromucosal spray) and its uses in various clinical trials. The article reported that the results from these clinical trials generally demonstrated "a reduction in the severity of the symptoms associated with spasticity." Spasticity is common in MS, involving muscles that stiffen and are difficult to move or control. Patients experienced a higher quality of life when they added Sativex to their treatment regimen. The profile concluded that "initial well-controlled studies with Sativex oromucosal spray administered as an add-on to usual therapy have produced promising results and highlight encouraging avenues for future research."

In a study published in 2013, Sativex was used to relieve symptoms of muscle spasticity. The fifteen-week-long double-blind, placebo-controlled trial involved 337 MS patients with spasticity. Results found that, compared with those who were treated with a placebo, 98 percent of patients treated with Sativex found some form of relief in the first four weeks of treatment. Any side effects from the Sativex dose were mild to moderate. The study's authors found that "Sativex treatment resulted in a significant reduction in treatment-resistant spasticity, in subjects with advanced MS and severe spasticity. The response observed within the first 4 weeks of treatment appears to be a useful aid to prediction of responder/non-responder status."

One of the leading researchers in CBD research, Dr. Zvi Vogel of Israel, helped write a 2011 study that demonstrated how CBD helped mice with MS symptoms. The mice had a condition similar to MS, in which their limbs were partially paralyzed. After being injected with CBD, the mice began to move and walk around again without limping. The CBD-treated group of mice had significantly less inflammation in their spinal cords than the untreated group. The CBD worked by stopping the mice's immune cells from attacking nerve cells in their spinal cords.

The Israeli researchers followed up this study with another study in 2013. In this study, the researchers isolated harmful immune cells from paralyzed mice. These immune cells had been harming the brains and spinal cords of the mice. Using THC and CBD, the researchers found that both of these compounds helped reduce the amount of inflammatory molecules being produced—in particular, an inflammatory molecule called interleukin 17 (IL-17), which is often indicated in MS cases. The study concluded that "the presence of CBD or THC restrains the immune cells from triggering the production of inflammatory molecules, and limits the molecules' ability to reach and damage the brain and spinal cord."

Hemp seed oil—which does not contain CBD or THC—has been shown in preliminary studies to be a possible treatment for MS symptoms because of its anti-inflammatory benefits. A 2012 study gathered twenty-three participants who were relapsing, remitting MS patients. They were given dosages of 18 to 21g per day of hemp seed oil and evening primrose oil in a 9-to-1 ratio for six months. In addition, patients were required to comply with a diet that included foods low in cholesterol and saturated/trans fats; a high amount of fruits, vegetables, nuts, seeds, fish, unrefined carbohydrates and olive or grape seed oils; and a reduction in sugar, refined starch, and food additives.

After six months of following the diet and consuming the hemp seed oil combination, the patients' blood was checked. Researchers found that the production of pro-inflammatory cytokines had significantly decreased, while production of anti-inflammatory cytokine IL-4 had blossomed. There was improvement in patients' expanded disability status scale (EDSS). The co-authors of the study concluded, "Our data demonstrated that co-supplemented hemp seed and evening primrose oils with...diet intervention may decrease the risk of developing MS related to the effects on decrease in pro-inflammatory and increase in anti-inflammatory cytokines."

How to Use: The cannabinoid drug Satevix is a 1:1 ratio of CBD and THC extracted from marijuana and approved around the world for the treatment of multiple sclerosis (MS) Self-medication in this population is ill advised and not recommended. If approved by the FDA here in the United States, Sativex prescriptions for a tested ration of CBD and THC for MS would only be available in pharmacies. Hemp seed oil with omega 3 ALA in addition to marine omega 3 EPA and DHA may enhance benefits.

NAUSEA AND VOMITING

While nausea is commonly triggered by a "stomach flu," it may be a symptom of a number of serious conditions and illnesses. Cannabidiol indirectly activates the receptor CB1 and other targets within the endocannabinoid system, thus regulating vomiting and nausea-like symptoms in a wide range of ailments. Research has proven it to be an effective antiemetic (anti-nausea/vomiting) treatment with fewer side effects than many drugs.

Although advocates of CBD are hopeful that CBD-rich hemp oil will soon become a widely accepted treatment for nausea and vomiting inducing conditions and illnesses, it is crucial that one does not self-medicate without a proper diagnosis and determining the cause of the nausea and vomiting.

How to Use: The FDA approved cannabinoid drugs from the 1980s for nausea and vomiting extracts or the extended half-life and longer relief of ingestible dietary supplements or edibles. CBDA may offer an alternative to those who cannot tolerate THC, while some report that CBD is more effective. Due to the large distribution of serotonin receptors in the gut, too much CBDA may actually cause nausea. It's about fine tuning so proceed slowly. Recommended dosage is 3 to 30 mg of CBDA or CBD taken daily. Check with your healthcare provider.

OPIATE ADDICTION

See ADDICTION, OPIATE.

PANIC ATTACK

See ANXIETY DISORDERS.

PMS

See **PREMENSTRUAL SYNDROME.**

POST TRAUMATIC STRESS DISORDER

See **ANXIETY DISORDERS.**

PREMENSTRUAL SYNDROME

If you are female, you have likely experienced premenstrual syndrome (PMS) at least once in your lifetime. It is characterized by a number of symptoms that generally appear one to two weeks before a woman menstruates. Although not a disease itself, PMS can be a painful and unpleasant experience. The symptoms can last anywhere from a day or two up to a week.

Symptoms that appear to be severe PMS may actually be indicative of another condition, such as endometriosis. A more severe form of PMS is PMDD, or Premenstrual Dysphoric Disorder. If you are experiencing intense PMS-like symptoms, it is best to speak with a doctor to determine if these symptoms are part of another condition.

Symptoms

Symptoms mostly include changes in mood, although some changes in physical appearance are noted. More than 200 symptoms have been linked with PMS. General symptoms include:

- Abdominal cramps
- Acne
- Anxiety
- Bloating
- Change in libido
- Depression
- Fatigue

- Food cravings
- Headache
- Irritability
- Lower back pain
- Mood swings

Triggers

The exact cause of PMS is unknown, although it is likely caused by hormonal changes that occur during the menstrual cycle. Symptoms can be worsened, but not caused, by poor diet or a pre-existing mood disorder, such as major depression disorder. Other risk factors include:

- Age: Women in their twenties through early forties are more likely to experience symptoms.
- Family history of depression
- Having at least one child
- High stress level

Conventional Treatment/Side Effects

There is not a "cure-all" for PMS, but many treatments are used with varying results. Lifestyle changes, such as eating a diet high in vitamins and minerals and low in sodium and exercising, can help reduce bloating and improve mood. Specifically, foods high in the substance tryptophan—such as turkey, milk, and bananas—can be beneficial, because tryptophan helps to build the hormone serotonin. Serotonin levels drop during PMS.

Medications that interact with hormones are sometimes used in more severe cases. For example, birth control pills may reduce symptoms in some women—but cause symptoms in other women. Antidepressant medications can be used in intervals to treat symptoms as they occur, although this may not be effective and can cause side effects.

Midol, an over-the-counter medication specifically targeting PMS symptoms (especially cramps), is a popular treatment. Other over-the-counter medications that are used to treat pain and cramps include aspirin and ibuprofen. At-home remedies can include using a heating pad to reduce cramps and pain; using essential oils, such as lavender, to reduce stress; and supplementing with calcium, magnesium, vitamin B6, and vitamin D.

CBD and Hemp Oil

CBD may be useful in managing PMS. In an article for the website Goop, Dr. Julie Holland described how CBD could benefit women struggling with PMS. CBD has anti-inflammatory, anti-anxiety, and muscle-relaxant properties. To exercise these effects, CBD interacts with the molecules in the endocannabinoid system responsible for managing stress and pain. The endocannabinoid system is made up of molecules that are similar to cannabis and help reduce stress and pain. The most significant of these molecules, anandamide, maintains balance in the hormonal and nervous systems; a higher anandamide level is linked with better stress management, according to Dr. Holland. Consuming CBD activates this endocannabinoid system to help bring the body back to a state of homeostasis.

The research focusing on PMS symptoms and cannabinoids has found that CBD "relaxes the mind and body" and "suppresses headaches and pain." In addition, the omega-6 and omega-3 fatty acids found in hemp seed oil are essential fats that help to regulate blood sugar levels, "fluctuations which are related to PMS."

How to Use: Recommended dosage is 3 to 30 mg of CBD and/or a CBDA-rich topical balm preparation taken daily. Check with your personal health-care provider. Raw hemp extracts with CBDA may also be effective. Hemp seed oil with omega 3 ALA in addition to marine omega 3 EPA and DHA may enhance benefits.

See **ANXIETY DISORDERS.**

SCHIZOPHRENIA

Schizophrenia is a mental illness in which a person experiences a distorted reality. The inability to think clearly, irrational behavior, and wildly varying emotions are all indicative of schizophrenia. Specifically, people with schizophrenia experience delusions, or thoughts that are not based in reality. They also often have visual or auditory hallucinations, especially hearing voices. Patients may be easily agitated or depressed, and may move and react oddly—for example, making excessive, useless movements. It is a critical, chronic condition that requires lifelong treatment to manage.

Symptoms

Schizophrenia symptoms can vary in their severity. In some patients, symptoms may always be present, while in others, symptoms get worse and then better. The disease usually starts to surface in your twenties. The following are the most common symptoms:

- Abnormal emotional responses
- Abnormal movements
- Delusions
- Disorganized thinking

- Hallucinations
- Hearing voices
- Loss of interest in hobbies
- Monotone speech

- Neglect of hygiene
- Social withdrawal

- Suicidal thoughts

Triggers

Although an exact cause has not been determined, schizophrenia is thought to be caused by a combination of genetics/family history, past psychoactive drug use, brain chemistry, and environment.

Conventional Treatment/Side Effects

In most cases, medication is necessary for managing schizophrenia. A class of drugs called antipsychotics are most often prescribed. They work on the dopamine neurotransmitter in the brain, which is responsible for managing emotions, movements, and generating pleasure. There are two types of antipsychotics. First-generation antipsychotics are less expensive than second-generation antipsychotics, but tend to have more severe side effects, including the possibility of developing a movement disorder. Both classes of antipsychotics block similar receptors in the brain.

Therapy and interventions may be effective in conjunction with prescription medicine. Such therapies can include individual therapy to teach patients to recognize abnormal thoughts and warning signs of a relapse; family therapy to extend support to patients' loved ones; and social skills training. In addition, many people with schizophrenia require at-home aides or case managers to help them take care of themselves and/or become employed.

CBD and Hemp Oil

High-THC cannabis can worsen symptoms of schizophrenia, especially anxiety and psychosis. CBD, on the other hand, cuts down these effects of THC.

A study published in the *Brazilian Journal of Medical and Biological Research* stated, "the antipsychotic-like properties of CBD have been investigated in animal models...which suggested that CBD has a pharmacological profile similar to atypical [second-generation] antipsychotic drugs."

According to a study conducted in the Illawarra Health and Medical Research Institute (IHMR), CBD "once isolated, could be used to treat negative cognitive symptoms of the severe mental illness – including social withdrawal and blunted emotional expression."

In another study led by Markus Leweke, University of Cologne in Germany, thirty-nine patients hospitalized for psychotic episodes were studied. Nineteen patients were treated with amisulpride, an antipsychotic medication, and the other twenty patients were given cannabidiol. Both groups showed a significant improvement in their symptoms at the end of the four-week trial. The patients taking CBD showed no difference from those taking amisulpride. Researchers concluded that CBD was not only on par with antipsychotic drugs in treating schizophrenia, but also free of the typical side effects associated with antipsychotics.

How to Use: Recommended dosage is 3 to 30 mg of CBD taken twice daily. Concentrated extracts may be most effective when combined with higher amounts of omega 3 EPA and DHA.

SKIN CONDISIONS

See **ECZEMA.**

THROMBOSIS

See **BLOOD CLOTS.**

THYROID DISORDER

See **HORMONAL IMBALANCE.**

ULCERATIVE COLITIS

Ulcerative colitis is a long-term inflammatory bowel disease causing inflammation and ulcers (sores) in the rectum and colon. The condition can be painful, embarrassing, and debilitating. It can affect people of all ages.

Symptoms

Symptoms may present themselves differently and progress differently in each person, however common symptoms may be:

- Abdominal pain
- Bloody stools
- Constipation
- Diarrhea, persistent
- Fever

- Frequent/urgent bowel movements
- Loss of appetite
- Mucus in stools
- Muscle aches
- Weight loss

Anxiety and stress may cause the symptoms to worsen.

Triggers

Ulcerative colitis may begin gradually and may worsen over time. The exact cause is unknown, but studies have indicated that the following factors may play a role in the condition.

- Heredity
- Environmental factors
- Over-active immune system

Although stress and diet are not causes, research has shown that they may increase the chances of flare-ups.

Conventional Treatment/Side Effects

Depending on the severity of the condition, certain anti-inflammatory drugs may be prescribed or surgery may be the option. Because some these drugs have severe side effects and because drugs that work for some may not work for other, it may take time to settle on a drug that helps you.

The drugs most commonly prescribed for this condition are aminosalicylates or corticosteroids. Antibiotics and immunosuppressant drugs may be prescribed as well. These drugs have a number of side effects, such as digestive distress, headaches, insomnia, and more serious side effects, for example high blood pressure, diabetes, osteoporosis, and a small risk of developing cancer.

CBD and Hemp Oil

Most research, thus far, has centered in studies using animals or biopsied human tissue. In a study cited in a 2011 issue of *PLOS ONE,* researchers studied "biopsies from individuals with ulcerative colitis" and found that "CBD was an effective anti-inflammatory agent, whether the biopsy was from a patient in remission or experiencing active disease." The researchers found that CBD affects certain cells that are the first line of defense against harmful pathogens. Normally, these cells stimulate inflammation in the GI tract by manufacturing a certain protein, whereas CBD modulates its production, therefore reducing inflammation.

Research suggests that CBD offers relief from symptoms of ulcerative colitis, such as pain relief, reduces nausea, and stimulates the appetite. In an article published in the October 2011 edition of *European Journal of Gastro-enterology & Hepatology*, the authors stated that cannabis is commonly used by IBD patients for symptom relief, in particular for those with a history of abdominal surgery and chronic abdominal pain.

How to Use: Recommended dosage is 3 to 30 mg of CBD taken twice daily. A combination of Raw CBDA rich hemp extracts with gold concentrated hemp extracts offer the widest possible range of cannabinoids in hemp. THC if tolerable may provide additional pain relief. Hemp seed oil with omega 3 ALA in addition to marine omega 3 EPA and DHA may enhance benefits.

See also: **CROHN'S DISEASE**

Resources

Unlike the resource centers for information on marijuana, resources for more information regarding hemp and hemp oil products are quite limited. Many of the hemp related websites are set up to sell products rather than focus on the research being conducted on hemp. We have tried to avoid including resources that sell hemp-related products. Please note all information below may be subject to change. It is therefore important to contact these centers before planning a visit.

CANNIBINOID THERAPY

CBD Resource Center

This resource center is a point of reference for recent studies, tests, or just general resources regarding CBD research and certain conditions.
https://blog.nectarleaf.com/cbd-resource-center/
1-415-935-1424

HEMP OIL RESOURCE GUIDE

Healthy Hemp Oil LTD

A resource that provides basic information that one should know about using and buying canabidiol, including benefits, current research, legal status, and the history of cannabidiol.
Office 3 Unit R
Penfold Works
Imperial Way
Watford, Herts United Kingdom, WD24 4YY
https://healthyhempoil.com/cannabidiol/
1-844-HEMPOIL (436-7645)

Hemp Business Journal

A newsletter that provides news and information primarily focused on the business of growing and selling industrial hemp and hemp products in the United States. In addition, it covers the science and politics affecting the hemp industry.
550 Larimer Street
Suite 123
Denver, Colorado 80202
www.hempbizjournal.com

Hemp Resource Center

This is a resource site that provides documentation, videos, and testimonials to help create a better understanding of hemp and how to use hemp products.
http://www.hempresourcecenter.org/
1-760-689-2151

Hemphasis

A website covering all aspects of hemp, including history, politics, science, products, and research.
www.hemphasis.net/Environment/environment.htm

Medical Jane

Medical Jane provides free medical cannabis education and resources to suffering patients. Provides a step-by-step patient guide to find optimal dosage and delivery method.
www.medicaljane.com/

Rick Simpson's Medicinal Hemp Oil

How to make Rick Simpson's medical help oil safely.
www.youtube.com/watch?v=KZXGH6mYr3Y

U.S. GOVERNMENT SITES
PROVIDING HEMP REGULATIONS

U.S. Government Hemp Film

Hemp for Victory (1942). View the original film produced and created by the Federal government during World War II to encourage farmers to grow hemp in the U.S. Shortly after the war, the government removed the film from its archives and deleted all official records indicating that this film had ever been produced.
www.globalhemp.com/1942/01/hemp-for-victory.html

State Industrial Hemp Statutes

NCSL provides laws and policies regarding industrial hemp as an agricultural commodity.
www.ncsl.org/research/agriculture-and-rural-development/state-industrial-hemp-statutes.aspx
United States Drug Enforcement Administration
The DEA provides news releases and clarifies the legal status of hemp and hemp products. DEA has 221 Domestic Offices in 21 Divisions throughout the U.S.
www.dea.gov/pubs/pressrel/pr100901.html

References

PART I. HEMP OIL AND CBD BASICS

CHAPTER I. THE HISTORY OF HEMP

Cannabis in Medical Practice: A Legal, Historical and Pharmacological Overview of the Therapeutic Use of Marijuana by Mary Lynn Mathre, R.N. (Michael Aldrich wrote Chapter 3; the info I provided is from page 35).

American Medical Association opposition to 1937 Act: Cary, EH. "Report of Committee on Legislative Activities," JAMA 108: 2214, 1937.

Axelrod and Hampson cannabinoid patent

http://patft.uspto.gov/netacgi/nph-Parser?Sect1=PTO1&Sect2=HITOFF&d=PALL&p=1&u=%2Fnetahtml%2FPTO%2Fsrchnum.htm&r=1&f=G&l=50&s1=6630507.PN.&OS=PN/6630507&RS=PN/6630507

https://bengreenfieldfitness.com/2015/06/how-to-use-cbd-oil/

www.cancer.gov/about-cancer/treatment/cam/patient/cannabis-pdq#section/all

www.cannalawblog.com/think-you-are-selling-legal-cbd-oil-dea-says-think-again/

Creation of Charlotte's Web CBD supplement

www.thekindpen.com/a-brief-history-of-medicinal-cbd-oil/

www.csdp.org/publicservice/anslinger.htm

Difference between hemp oil and CBD oil

www.chronictherapy.co/hemp-oil-vs-cbd-oil-whats-the-difference-2

Difference between CBD and THC structures

https://cbdoilreview.org/cbd-cannabidiol/thc-cbd/

http://druglibrary.org/schaffer/hemp/history/first12000/3.htm

The Emperor Wears No Clothes by Jack Herer, 1985

www.mit.edu/~thistle/v13/2/history.html

Epidiolex research and seizures

http://dev-gwpharma.pantheonsite.io/about-us/news/gw-pharmaceuticals
-announces-second-positive-phase-3-pivotal-trial-epidiolex

http://extract.suntimes.com/news/10/153/15944/fda-issues-warning-letters-to-canna-
bis-cbd-companies

www.federalregister.gov/documents/2016/12/14/2016-29941/establishment-of-a-new
-drug-code-for-marihuana-extract

GW Pharmaceuticals history

www.gwpharm.com/about-us/history-approach

The Health Effects of Cannabis and Cannabinoids, Board on Population Health and Public

Health Practice; Health and Medicine Division; National Academies of Sciences, Engineering,
and Medicine, The National Academies Press, 2017. www.nap.edu/24625

www.napwww.hort.purdue.edu/newcrop/ncnu02/v5-284.html

Mechoulam discoveries about CBD

www.projectcbd.org/sites/projectcbd/files/downloads/mechoulam-iacm-07.pdf

www.mountvernon.org/education/primary-sources-2/article/george-washington-letter
-to-james-gildart/

www.mountvernon.org/george-washington/the-man-the-myth/george-washington-grew
-hemp

www.ncbi.nlm.nih.gov/pubmed/23278122

www.ncsl.org/research/agriculture-and-rural-development/state-industrial-hemp-statutes.aspx

www.pbs.org/wgbh/pages/frontline/shows/dope/interviews/musto.html

www.pbs.org/wgbh/pages/frontline/shows/dope/etc/cron.html

www.politico.com/magazine/story/2015/01/drug-war-the-hunting-of-billie-holiday-
114298?o=0 – excerpt from *Chasing The Scream: The First and Last Days of the War on Drugs* by
Johann Hari

Roger Adams article about CBD isolation

http://chemistry.mdma.ch/hiveboard/rhodium/pdf/cannabidiol.structure.pdf

www.smithsonianmag.com/history/uncovering-the-truth-behind-the-myth-of-pancho-villa-
movie-star-110349996/

Structure of CBD

https://pubchem.ncbi.nlm.nih.gov/compound/cannabidiol#section=Top

Structure of THC

https://pubchem.ncbi.nlm.nih.gov/compound/16078#section=Top

www.ukcia.org/research/potnight/pn4.htm

1619 Virginia Assembly Law: http://oll.libertyfund.org/pages/1619-laws-enacted-by-the-first
-general-assembly-of-virginia

https://en.wikipedia.org/wiki/Harry_J._Anslinger#The_campaign_against_marijuana_1930.
E2.80.931937

CHAPTER 2. THE SCIENCE OF CBD

Animal study with CBD and 5-HT1A

www.ncbi.nlm.nih.gov/pubmed/24923339

Cannabinoid receptors—what they are and what they do www.ncbi.nlm.nih.gov/pmc/articles/PMC2931548/http://onlinelibrary.wiley.com/doi/10.1111/j.1365-2826.2008.01671.x/full

CBD and GABA

www.ncbi.nlm.nih.gov/pubmed/28249817

CBD and TRPV-1

www.ncbi.nlm.nih.gov/pmc/articles/PMC1575333/

CBD and turmeric

https://bengreenfieldfitness.com/2015/06/how-to-use-cbd-oil/

CBD interactions with enzymes

www.projectcbd.org/article/cbd-drug-interactions-role-cytochrome-p450

DEA talking points with Congress

www.naihc.org/member-links/323-us-drug-enforcement-administration-dea-hemp-talking-points

https://elixinol.com/blog/how-does-cannabidiol-cbd-work/

The Emperor Wears No Clothes by Jack Herer

http://jackherer.com.s216995.gridserver.com/emperor-3/

Explaining how CBD works on different receptors—CB1 receptor

www.beyondthc.com/wp-content/uploads/2012/07/CBDiary21.pdf

United States Farm bill

www.votehemp.com/2014_farm_bill_section_7606.html

GPR55 and CBDs and osteoclasts

www.ncbi.nlm.nih.gov/pmc/articles/PMC2737440/

The Health Effects of Cannabis and Cannabinoids, Board on Population Health and Public

Health Practice; Health and Medicine Division; National Academies of Sciences, Engineering, and Medicine, The National Academies Press, 2017. www.nap.edu/24625

Hemp seed benefits/grossamide

www.ncbi.nlm.nih.gov/pubmed/28224333?dopt=Abstract

Hemp vs. marijuana

http://sites.miis.edu/thinkhempythoughts/hemp-vs-marijuana/ AND www.legvi.org/CommiteeMeetings/31st%20Legislature%20Committees/COMMITTEE%20OF%20RULES%20&%20JUDICIARY/2016/February%2017th/Bill%20No.%2031-0100/Difference%20between%20Hemp%20and%20Marijuana.pdf

How Does Cannabidiol work inside the body (with references) – discusses cannabinoid receptors in the body

www.medicinalgenomics.com/wp-content/uploads/2013/01/Bergamaschi_2011.pdf

www.nateralife.com/blog/lifestyle/omega-truth-hemp-vs-fish-oil/

www.projectcbd.org/how-cbd-works

Safety of CBD

www.safeaccessnow.org

Simple explanation of the endocannabinoid system and cell receptors http://herb.co/2016/07/28/endocannabinoid-system-dummies/

What are cannabinoid receptors?

www.massroots.com/learn/what-are-cannabinoid-receptors

CHAPTER 3. LEGAL STATUS OF HEMP AND CBD OIL

Mead, Alice. "The legal status of cannabis (marijuana) and cannabidiol (CBD) under U.S. law." *Epilepsy and Behavior*, 2017.

CBD effect on addiction

www.ncbi.nlm.nih.gov/pmc/articles/PMC4444130/

Conclusions from LaGuardia committee

www.druglibrary.net/schaffer/Library/studies/lag/conc1.htm

Drug schedules

www.dea.gov/druginfo/ds.shtml

www.federalregister.gov/documents/2016/08/12/2016-19146/statement-of-principles-on-industrial-hemp

www.federalregister.gov/documents/2016/12/14/2016-29941/establishment-of-a-new-drug-code-for-marihuana-extract

www.forbes.com/sites/daviddisalvo/2016/12/31/states-with-medical-marijuana-laws-have-fewer-traffic-fatalities-but-why-isnt-clear/#43691f5155c8

Harrison Act

www.druglibrary.org/schaffer/library/studies/cu/cu8.html

HIA vs DEA

www.rollingstone.com/culture/features/hemp-wars-inside-the-fight-for-federally-legal-cbd-w477379

History and overview of industrial hemp

http://maui.hawaii.edu/hooulu/2016/01/15/industrial-hemp-a-history-and-overview-of
-the-super-crop-and-its-trillion-dollar-future/

How did Marijuana become illegal in the first place?

www.drugpolicy.org/blog/how-did-marijuana-become-illegal-first-place

Leary vs US

https://supreme.justia.com/cases/federal/us/395/6/

Marijuana curbing opioid addiction

www.nbcnews.com/health/health-news/legalized-marijuana-could-help-curb-opioid-epi-
demic-study-finds-n739301

Marijuana and violent crime

www.ncbi.nlm.nih.gov/pmc/articles/PMC3966811/

www.naihc.org/hemp_information/content/hemp.mj.html

www.projectcbd.org/article/sourcing-cbd-marijuana-industrial-hemp-vagaries-federal-law

Proposed Industrial Hemp Farming Act

www.votehemp.com/PR/2015-1-22-congress-introduces-hemp-farming-acts.html

Research obstacles

www.nytimes.com/2014/08/10/us/politics/medical-marijuana-research-hits-the-wall
-of-federal-law.html

www.reuters.com/article/us-health-marijuana-traffic-death-idUSKBN14H1LQ

State marijuana laws

http://norml.org/laws

Timeline of marijuana laws

www.pbs.org/wgbh/pages/frontline/shows/dope/etc/cron.html

Traffic and marijuana study

http://norml.org/news/2013/08/15/study-passage-of-medical-marijuana-laws-associat-
ed-with-reduced-incidences-of-alcohol-related-traffic-fatalities

Transcript of *Hemp for Victory* movie

www.globalhemp.com/1942/01/hemp-for-victory.html

USDA and DEA clarify the farm bill

www.congress.gov/bill/114th-congress/senate-bill/134

CHAPTER 4. A BUYER'S GUIDE

Alice Mead, J.D. Ll.M *Epilepsy & Behavior*, November 2016, www.epilepsybehavior.com/
article/S1525-5050(16)30585-6/pdf

CBD User's Manual

www.projectcbd.org/guidance/cbd-users-manual

PART 2. HEALING WITH HEMP OIL

ADDICTION, OPIATE

Gaviria M. *Chasing Heroi*. Frontline, 2016. *The Health Effects of Cannabis and Cannabinoids,* Board on Population Health and Public Health Practice; Health and Medicine Division; National Academies of Sciences, Engineering, and Medicine, The National Academies Press, 2017. www.nap.edu/24625

Katsidoni V, Anagnostou I, Panagis G. Cannabidiol inhibits the reward-facilitating effect of morphine: involvement of 5-HT1A receptors in the dorsal raphe nucleus. *Addict Biol.* 2013;18(2):286-296.

Ren Y, Whittard J, Higuera-Matas A, Morris CV, Hurd YL. Cannabidiol, a nonpsychotropic component of cannabis, inhibits cue-induced heroin seeking and normalizes discrete mesolimbic neuronal disturbances. *J Neurosci.* 2009;29(47):14764–14769.

Sulak, Dustin. "America's Opiate Crisis: How Medical Cannabis Can Help"

www.projectcbd.org/article/americas-opiate-crisis-how-medical-cannabis-can-help

Causes

http://opium.com/addiction/12-common-triggers-for-opiate-addicts/

CBD USE

https://cannabistraininguniversity.com/opioid-withdrawal-and-cbd/

OPIATE ABUSE

http://drugabuse.com/library/opiate-abuse/

Treatment

www.everydayhealth.com/news/drugs-that-work-opioid-addiction-treatment/

Treatment

www.marijuanadoctors.com/blog/medical-marijuana/marijuana-treatment-for-opiate-addiction

AGE-RELATED MACULAR DEGENERATION

Haddrill; Marilyn. "Macular Degeneration Treatment"

https://maculacenter.com/eye-procedures/avastin/

Cannabinoid uses

www.medicalmarijuana.com/medical-marijuana-treatments-cannabis-uses/md-and-cannabinoids/

Cannabis and Macular Degeneration: Can It Help?

https://unitedpatientsgroup.com/blog/2016/10/30/cannabis-macular-degeneration

Symptoms

www.webmd.com/eye-health/macular-degeneration/age-related-macular-degeneration
-symptoms

Treatments

www.allaboutvision.com/conditions/amd-treatments.htm

ALZHEIMER'S DISEASE

Cheng D, Spiro AS, Jenner AM, Garner B, Karl T. "Long-term cannabidiol treatment prevents the development of social recognition memory deficits in Alzheimer's disease transgenic mice." *Journal of Alzheimers Disease*. 2014;42(4):1383-96. doi: 10.3233/JAD-140921.

"The Effects of Medical Marijuana on Alzheimer's Treatment" *Journal of Alzheimer's Disease*. December 7, 2016.

www.alzheimers.net/6-15-15-effects-of-medical-marijuana-on-alzheimers/

Ellison, James M., MD, MPH. "Possible Causes of Alzheimer's Disease"

www.alz.org/research/science/major_milestones_in_alzheimers.asp

The Health Effects of Cannabis and Cannabinoids, Board on Population Health and Public

Health Practice; Health and Medicine Division; National Academies of Sciences, Engineering, and Medicine, The National Academies Press, 2017. www.nap.edu/24625

Causes

www.brightfocus.org/alzheimers/article/possible-causes-alzheimers-disease

www.greenmedinfo.com/blog/marijuana-compound-found-superior-drugs-alzheimers

Hemp oil

https://healthyhempoil.com/alzheimers-cbd/

Symptoms

http://health.facty.com/conditions/alzheimers/10-symptoms-of-alzheimer/10/

Symptoms

www.mayoclinic.org/diseases-conditions/alzheimers-disease/symptoms-causes/
dxc-20167103

ANXIETY DISORDERS

Blessing EM, Steenkamp MM, Manzanares J, Marmar CR. "Cannabidiol as a Potential Treatment for Anxiety Disorders" *Neurotherapeutics*. 2015;12(4):825–36.

Grohol John M, Psy.D. "Anxiety Disorders" https://psychcentral.com/disorders/anxiety/

The Health Effects of Cannabis and Cannabinoids, Board on Population Health and Public Health Practice; Health and Medicine Division; National Academies of Sciences, Engineering, and Medicine, The National Academies Press, 2017. www.nap.edu/24625

Kossen, Jeremy." How Cannabidiol (CBD) Works for Treating Anxiety" www.leafly.com/
news/health/cbd-for-treating-anxiety

Cannibinoid study

www.cannabisreports.com/cannabis-studies/cannabidiol-induces-rapid-acting-antidepressant-like-effects-and-enhances-cortical-5-htglutamate-neurotransmission-role-of-5-ht1a-receptors

Drugs

www.rxlist.com/anxiety_medications-page4/drugs-condition.htm

APPETITE LOSS

Sircus, Mark. *Healing With Medical Marijuana.* Square One Publishers: Garden City Park, New York, 2017.

The Health Effects of Cannabis and Cannabinoids, Board on Population Health and Public

Health Practice; Health and Medicine Division; National Academies of Sciences, Engineering, and Medicine, The National Academies Press, 2017. www.nap.edu/24625

CBD benefits

https://cbdoilreview.org/cbd-cannabidiol/cbd-benefits/

www.ilovegrowingmarijuana.com/appetite/

www.medicinenet.com/appendicitis_quiz/quiz.htm

ARTHRITIS

Sircus, Mark. *Healing With Medical Marijuana.* Square One Publishers: Garden City Park, New York, 2017.

Butterfield, Delilah. "Can Arthritis Pain & Inflammation Be Treated With Cannabis?" August 6, 2016

SWC Team. "Medical Cannabis Can Help Arthritis Patients" September 11, 2015

http://blog.swcarizona.com/blog/author/swc-team

CBD benefits

http://thehempoilbenefits.com/cbd-oil-rheumatoid-arthritis

http://herb.co/2016/08/06/arthritis-pain-inflammation/

www.medicalnewstoday.com/articles/7621.php

ATTENTION DEFICIT HYPERACTIVITY DISORDER

Bearman, David, MD. "Cannabis Efficacy in Treating ADD & ADHD." http://inorml.com/blog/2012/08/05/cannabis-efficacy-in-treating-add-adhd-david-bearman-md/

Brosious, Emily Gray. "Could this medical marijuana tincture become the new go-to ADHD treatment?"

http://extract.suntimes.com/extract-news/medical-marijuana-tincture-add-adhd-treatment-cbd-mendo-focus/

Darby Damien. "ADHD and CBD (How About the Hemp Option?"

www.hempforfitness.com/2016/02/01/adhd-and-cbd/

Grohol, J. (2017). "Causes of Adult Attention Deficit Hyperactivity Disorder (ADHD)". *PsychCentral.*

https://psychcentral.com/disorders/adhd/causes-of-adult-attention-deficit-hyperactivity
-disorder-adhd/

Causes

https://psychcentral.com/disorders/adhd/causes-of-adult-attention-deficit-hyperactivity
-disorder-adhd/

Data and Statistics

www.help4adhd.org/Understanding-ADHD/About-ADHD/Data-and-Statistics.aspx

http://intranet.tdmu.edu.ua/data/kafedra/internal/nervous_desease/classes_stud/en/med/
lik/ptn/psihyatry/4/10%20Behavioral%20disorders%20which%20start%20in%20child.htm

Pediatric Cannabis Support

http://pediatriccannabissupport.com/startingyourchildonmedicalmarijuana/

Treatment

https://psychcentral.com/disorders/adhd/treatment-for-attention-deficit-hyperactivity-dis-
order-adhd/

BLOOD CLOTS

Gerber, Jeandre. "Using Medical Marijuana with Blood thinners—What to Know." *Medical
Marijuana Research,* June, 28, 2015.

Causes

http://health.facty.com/ailments/bood-clot/10-causes-of-blood-clots/10/

www.mayoclinic.org/symptoms/blood-clots/basics/causes/sym-20050850

Research

www.marijuanadoctors.com/blog/medical-marijuana-research/using-medical-marijuana
-with-blood-thinners-what-to-know

Symptoms

www.healthline.com/health/how-to-tell-if-you-have-a-blood-clot#overview1

www.webmd.com/dvt/blood-clot-symptoms

Treatment

www.stoptheclot.org/learn_more/blood_clot_treatment.htm

www.rxlist.com/heparin-side-effects-drug-center.htm

CANCER

Journal of the National Cancer Institute Advance Access on December 25th of 2007 in a paper enti-
tled "Inhibition of Cancer Cell Invasion by Cannabinoids via Increased Expression of Tissue
Inhibitor of Matrix Metalloproteinases." December 25, 2007.

The Health Effects of Cannabis and Cannabinoids, Board on Population Health and Public Health
Practice; Health and Medicine Division; National Academies of Sciences, Engineering, and
Medicine, The National Academies Press, 2017. www.nap.edu/24625

Limebeer, C.L., and Parker, L.A. (1999, December 16). "Delta-9-tetrahydrocannabinol interferes with the establishment and the expression of conditioned rejection reactions produced by cyclophosphamide: a rat model of nausea." *Neuroreport*, 10(19), 3769-72. Retrieved from http://journals.lww.com/neuroreport/pages/articleviewer. aspx?year=1999&issue=12160&article=00009&type=abstract.

Mechoulam, R., and Hanus, L. (2001). "The cannabinoids: An overview. Therapeutic implications in vomiting and nausea after cancer chemotherapy, in appetite promotion, in multiple sclerosis and in neuroprotection." *Pain Research and Management*, 6(2), 67-73. Retrieved from http://downloads.hindawi.com/journals/prm/2001/183057.pdf.

Sircus, Mark. *Healing With Medical Marijuana*. Square One Publishers, Garden City: New York, 2017.

National Cancer Institute www.cancer.gov/about-cancer/understanding/what-is-cancer

Causes

https://en.wikipedia.org/wiki/Cancer#Causes

Effects

www.medicalmarijuanainc.com/chemotherapy-side-effects-medical-marijuana-research -overview/

Symptoms

www.cancercenter.com/terms/cancer-symptoms/

www.emedicinehealth.com/cancer_symptoms/page2_em.htm

CROHN'S DISEASE

Butterfield, Delilah. "Will Cannabis Help Send Crohn's Disease Into Remission?" October 25, 2016. http://herb.co/2016/10/25/cannabis-crohns-disease-remission/

Overview

www.mayoclinic.org/diseases-conditions/crohns-disease/basics/definition/CON-20032061

www.stelarainfo.com/crohns-disease/overview/what-is-crohns-disease?&utm_source= bing&utm_medium=cpc&utm_campaign=CD+Condition+-+Phrase%2FExact&utm_content =CD+General&utm_term=crohns+disease&gclid=COj20oOBsdQCFURLgQodeM8Dsw& gclsrc=ds

Research

https://blog.endoca.com/news/recent-research-showed-cbd-colitis-might-cure/

Symptoms

www.webmd.com/ibd-crohns-disease/crohns-disease/tc/crohns-disease-symptoms

DEPRESSION

Butterfield, Delilah. "How Cannabis Treats Depression." June 3, 2016. http://herb. co/2016/06/26/mind-4-cannabis-fights-depression/

The Health Effects of Cannabis and Cannabinoids, Board on Population Health and Public Health Practice; Health and Medicine Division; National Academies of Sciences, Engineering, and Medicine, The National Academies Press, 2017. www.nap.edu/24625

Diagnosis

www.depressiontoolkit.org/aboutyourdiagnosis/depression.asp

www.mentalhealth.fitness/learn-about-your-diagnosis/depression

Effects

http://extract.suntimes.com/extract-news/study-cbd-cannabinoid-marijuana-induces-anti-depressant-like-effects/

www.nimh.nih.gov/health/topics/depression/index.shtml

Treatment

https://healthyhempoil.com/cbd-depression/

www.livescience.com/34718-depression-treatment-psychotherapy-anti-depressants.html

https://psychcentral.com/disorders/depression/depression-treatment/3/

DIABETES

Butterfield, Delilah . "Does Cannabis Help With Diabetes Treatment?" September 6, 2016. http://herb.co/2016/09/06/cannabis-help-diabetes/

"CBD compound in cannabis could treat diabetes, researchers suggest." Fri, 24 Apr 2015

www.diabetes.co.uk/news/2015/Apr/cbd-compound-in-cannabis-could-treat-diabetes,-researchers-suggest-95335970.html

Leontis, Lisa M. RN, ANP-C and Hess-Fischl, Amy MS, RD, LDN, BC-ADM, CDE. "Type 2 Diabetes Causes: Genetics and Lifestyle Choices Play a Role."

www.endocrineweb.com/conditions/type-2-diabetes/type-2-diabetes-causes

Benefits

https://sensiseeds.com/en/blog/top-5-benefits-cannabis-diabetes/

Overview

www.medicalnewstoday.com/info/diabetes

https://medlineplus.gov/diabetes.html

www.webmd.com/diabetes/ss/slideshow-insulin-resistance

Treatment

www.diabetes.co.uk/features/diabetes-medication-side-effects.html

http://drsircus.com/diabetes/cannabidiol-and-magnesium-help-treats-diabetes/

http://idweeds.com/cbd-diabetes-treatment/

ECZEMA

Research

www.finola.fi/FinolaOilandAtopy.pdf

www.naturalnews.com/036039_hemp_seeds_oil_EFAs.html

Symptoms

www.mayoclinic.org/diseases-conditions/eczema/basics/symptoms/con-20032073

Treatment

http://eczemafree.org/95/conventional-medical-treatments-of-eczema-and-their-side
-effects/

www.huffingtonpost.com/maria-rodale/9-ways-to-use-hemp-oil-in_b_10145990.html

www.webmd.com/skin-problems-and-treatments/guide/atopic-dermatitis-eczema#1

www.medicaljane.com/2014/12/24/the-beauty-of-hemp-seed-oil/

EPILEPSY

Clabria, Stephen. "American Epilepsy Society Just Confirmed CBD Stops Epileptic Seizures."
February 22, 2017. http://herb.co/2017/02/22/american-epilepsy-society-cbd/

The Health Effects of Cannabis and Cannabinoids, Board on Population Health and Public Health
Practice; Health and Medicine Division; National Academies of Sciences, Engineering, and
Medicine, The National Academies Press, 2017. www.nap.edu/24625

Preidt, Robert. "Pot Ingredient Might Ease Severe Epilepsy" *Health Day News*, April, 18, 2017.

Research

www.cureepilepsy.org/research/cbd-and-epilepsy.asp

Symptoms

www.epilepsy.com/learn/seizures-youth/about-kids/signs-symptoms

www.mayoclinic.org/diseases-conditions/epilepsy/symptoms-causes/dxc-20117207

www.webmd.com/epilepsy/tc/epilepsy-symptoms#1

Treatment

www.webmd.com/epilepsy/news/20170418/pot-ingredient-might-ease-severe-epilepsy#1

FIBROMYALGIA

Causes

www.mayoclinic.org/diseases-conditions/fibromyalgia/symptoms-causes/dxc-20317796

Treatment

www.fibromyalgiatreating.com/cbd-oil-fibromyalgia-treatment/

www.healthline.com/health/fibromyalgi

www.medicinenet.com/script/main/art.asp?articlekey=89309&page=1#what_is_
fibromyalgia

GLAUCOMA

Boyd, Kierstan. "What Is Glaucoma?" March 1, 2017.

www.aao.org/eye-health/diseases/what-is-glaucoma

European Journal of Neuroscience. "The synthetic cannabinoid WIN55212-2 decreases the intraocular pressure in human glaucoma resistant to conventional therapies." January 2001

http://onlinelibrary.wiley.com/wol1/doi/10.1046/j.0953-816X.2000.01401.x/full

Graefe's Archive for Clinical and Experimental Ophthalmology. "A submicron emulsion of HU-211, a synthetic cannabinoid, reduces intraocular pressure in rabbits." April 2000.

https://link.springer.com/article/10.1007%2Fs004170050361

The Health Effects of Cannabis and Cannabinoids, Board on Population Health and Public Health Practice; Health and Medicine Division; National Academies of Sciences, Engineering, and Medicine, The National Academies Press, 2017. www.nap.edu/24625

Causes/Symptoms

www.webmd.com/eye-health/glaucoma-eyes

Dosage

https://cbdoilreview.org/cbd-cannabidiol/cbd-dosage/

www.mayoclinic.org/diseases-conditions/glaucoma/basics/treatment/con-20024042

Treatment

www.aao.org/eye-health/diseases/glaucoma-treatment

www.glaucomafoundation.org/treating_glaucoma.htm

HEADACHE

Causes

www.health.com/health/gallery/0,,20484672,00.html#tension-headaches-1

Symptoms

www.mayoclinic.org/diseases-conditions/migraine-headache/symptoms.../dxc-20202434

Treatment

www.endoca.com/blog/cbd/cbd-for-migraines-headaches/

http://thehempoilbenefits.com/cbd-for-migraines

http://mynaturalmigrainetreatments.com/hemp-oil-and-migraine/

www.webmd.com/migraines-headaches/news/.../migraine-drugs-effects-scare-many-awa...

HEART DISEASE

British Journal of Clinical Pharmacology. "Is the cardiovascular system a therapeutic target for cannabidiol?" February, 2013.

Supplyside Insider. "The Essential Debate: The Balance Between Omega-6 and Omega-3." February, 2013.

Overview

http://ajpheart.physiology.org/content/293/6/H3602.long

www.cdc.gov/dhdsp/data_statistics/fact_sheets/fs_heart_disease.htm

www.drugs.com/warfarin.html

www.mayoclinic.org/diseases-conditions/heart-disease/basics/definition/con-20034056

Research

www.ncbi.nlm.nih.gov/pmc/articles/PMC3579247/

www.projectcbd.org/heart-disease

Treatment

www.mayoclinic.org/diseases-conditions/high-blood-pressure/in-depth/ace-inhibitors/art-20047480?pg=2

https://medlineplus.gov/bloodthinners.html

http://undergroundhealthreporter.com/hempseed-oil-health-benefits-from-heart-disease-to-dementia-prevention/

www.webmd.com/heart-disease/common-medicine-heart-disease-patients#1

HIGH BLOOD PRESSURE

www.heart.org/HEARTORG/Conditions/HighBloodPressure/KnowYourNumbers/Understanding-Blood-Pressure-Readings_UCM_301764_Article.jsp#.WUlsFtQrJpg

www.heart.org/HEARTORG/Conditions/HighBloodPressure/UnderstandSymptomsRisks/What-are-the-Symptoms-of-High-Blood-Pressure_UCM_301871_Article.jsp#.WRCpY9Lyu1s

Overview

www.leafly.com/news/health/cannabis-high-blood-pressure-hypertension

Research

www.ncbi.nlm.nih.gov/pmc/articles/PMC3579247/

Treatment

www.mayoclinic.org/diseases-conditions/high-blood-pressure/basics/treatment/con-20019580

www.mayoclinic.org/diseases-conditions/high-blood-pressure/in-depth/ace-inhibitors/art-20047480?pg=2

www.medicalmarijuana.com/medical-marijuana-treatments-cannabis-uses/cannabinoids-lower-blood-pressure-to-normal-levels/

www.webmd.com/heart-disease/guide/heart-disease-calcium-channel-blocker-drugs#1-4

HIGH CHOLESTEROL

Causes

www.mayoclinic.org/diseases-conditions/high-blood-cholesterol/symptoms-causes/dxc-20181874

www.nhlbi.nih.gov/health/resources/heart/heart-cholesterol-hbc-what-html

Research

www.researchgate.net/publication/51089800_The_Non-Psychoactive_Plant_Cannabinoid_Cannabidiol_Affects_Cholesterol_Metabolism-Related_Genes_in_Microglial_Cells

www.webmd.com/cholesterol-management/tc/high-cholesterol-overview#1

Symptoms

www.healthline.com/health/high-cholesterol-symptoms

www.mayoclinic.org/diseases-conditions/high-blood-cholesterol/symptoms-causes/dxc-20181874

Treatment

http://articles.mercola.com/sites/articles/archive/2016/02/10/5-reasons-why-you-should-not-take-statins.aspx

www.livestrong.com/article/420062-cholesterol-control-with-hemp-oil/

www.webmd.com/cholesterol-management/news/20140818/statins-side-effects-news#1

www.zliving.com/wellness/natural-remedies/9-health-benefits-of-hemp-oil-that-you-should-know

HORMONE IMBALANCE

Research

http://ajcn.nutrition.org/content/54/4/684.short

http://fhcobwomenshealth.com/hormone-imbalance.php

www.ncbi.nlm.nih.gov/pubmed/15385858

Treatment

www.livestrong.com/article/176729-drugs-for-hormonal-imbalance/

www.mayoclinic.org/diseases-conditions/high-blood-pressure/in-depth/ace-inhibitors/art-20047480?pg=2

https://discovercbd.com/blogs/cbd-news/hemp-and-hormones

Symptoms

www.webmd.com/women/ss/slideshow-hormone-imbalance

INFLAMMATION

"Cannabinoids as novel anti-inflammatory drugs." October 2009.

www.ncbi.nlm.nih.gov/pmc/articles/PMC2828614/

Research Gate. "Anti-inflammatory ω-3 endocannabinoid epoxides." July 2017.ωω

Causes/Symptoms

www.livescience.com/52344-inflammation.html

www.medicalnewstoday.com/articles/248423.php?

www.prevention.com/health/signs-chronic-inflammation

www.webmd.com/arthritis/about-inflammation#1-4

Treatment

https://elixinol.com/blog/cannabinoids-can-stop-inflammation/

www.mayoclinic.org/steroids/art-20045692

https://pdfs.semanticscholar.org/4b5c/e865d8f85e86e250715c6e716a4fcc4c8844.pdf

INSOMNIA

The Health Effects of Cannabis and Cannabinoids, Board on Population Health and Public Health Practice; Health and Medicine Division; National Academies of Sciences, Engineering, and Medicine, The National Academies Press, 2017. www.nap.edu/24625

Research

www.projectcbd.org/sleep-disorders

www.tandfonline.com/doi/full/10.1080/14728222.2017.1353603

https://en.wikipedia.org/wiki/Sleep_onset_latency

Symptoms/Causes

www.mayoclinic.org/diseases-conditions/insomnia/home/ovc-20256955

www.webmd.com/sleep-disorders/guide/insomnia-symptoms-and-causes#1

www.webmd.com/sleep-disorders/guide/sleep-disorders-symptoms-types

Treatment

https://elixinol.com/blog/how-does-cannabidiol-affect-sleep-and-insomnia/

www.mayoclinic.org/diseases-conditions/insomnia/diagnosis-treatment/treatment/txc-20256979

www.mayoclinic.org/diseases-conditions/sleep-apnea/basics/definition/con-20020286

IRRITABLE BOWEL SYNDROME

Overview

www.medicinenet.com/irritable_bowel_syndrome_ibs/article.htm

The Health Effects of Cannabis and Cannabinoids, Board on Population Health and Public Health Practice; Health and Medicine Division; National Academies of Sciences, Engineering, and Medicine, The National Academies Press, 2017. www.nap.edu/24625

Research

www.ncbi.nlm.nih.gov/pubmed/24977967

Symptoms/Causes

www.emedicinehealth.com/irritable_bowel_syndrome/page3_em.htm#what_medications_treat_irritable_bowel_syndrome_ibs_symptoms

www.mayoclinic.org/diseases-conditions/irritable-bowel-syndrome/basics/definition/con-20024578

Treatment

https://aboutibs.org/what-is-ibs-sidenav/treatments-for-ibs.html

http://cbdcentral.org/cbd-conditions/irritable-bowel-syndrome-ibs/

www.crescolabs.com/conditions/irritable-bowel-syndrome/

https://thehempdoctor.co.uk/cbd-oil-blog/cbd-oil-and-irritable-bowel-syndrome-ibs-/?sl=en

http://herb.co/2016/11/15/irritable-bowel-syndrome/

www.mayoclinic.org/diseases-conditions/irritable-bowel-syndrome/basics/treatment/con-20024578

www.niddk.nih.gov/health-information/digestive-diseases/irritable-bowel-syndrome/treatment

www.webmd.com/drugs/2/drug-4789-4025/loperamide-oral/loperamide-oral/details

MULTIPLE SCLEROSIS (MS)

Overview

The Health Effects of Cannabis and Cannabinoids, Board on Population Health and Public Health Practice; Health and Medicine Division; National Academies of Sciences, Engineering, and Medicine, The National Academies Press, 2017. www.nap.edu/24625

Symptoms/Causes

www.abovems.com/en_us/home/ms101/symptoms/most-common-ms-symptoms.html

www.mayoclinic.org/diseases-conditions/multiple-sclerosis/symptoms-causes/dxc-20131884

www.nationalmssociety.org/What-is-MS/What-Causes-MS

Treatment

www.endoca.com/blog/news/new-hope-multiple-sclerosis-cannabidiol/

www.mayoclinic.org/diseases-conditions/multiple-sclerosis/diagnosis-treatment/treatment/txc-20131903

Research

www.ncbi.nlm.nih.gov/pmc/articles/PMC3648912/

www.ncbi.nlm.nih.gov/pubmed/21456949

www.ncbi.nlm.nih.gov/pubmed/23892791

www.projectcbd.org/multiple-sclerosis-ms

www.tandfonline.com/doi/abs/10.1179/016164109X12590518685660

www.tandfonline.com/doi/abs/10.1586/ern.11.47?journalCode=iern20

NAUSEA AND VOMITING

British Journal of Pharmacology. Parker, LA, et al. "Regulation of nausea and vomiting by cannabinoids." August 1, 2011.

The Health Effects of Cannabis and Cannabinoids, Board on Population Health and Public Health Practice; Health and Medicine Division; National Academies of Sciences, Engineering, and Medicine, The National Academies Press, 2017. www.nap.edu/24625

Causes

www.healthline.com/health/nausea-and-vomiting#overview1

www.mayoclinic.org/symptoms/nausea/basics/causes/sym-20050736

www.webmd.com/digestive-disorders/digestive-diseases-nausea-vomiting

Research/Treatment

www.catscientific.com/therapeutic-effects-cbd-nausea-vomiting/

www.cbdpure.com/nausea.html

www.hempoilfacts.com/cannabidiol-cbd-nausea-research/

http://herb.co/2017/02/28/cannabis-treat-nausea/

www.ncbi.nlm.nih.gov/pubmed/21175589

PREMENSTRUAL SYNDROME

Symptoms/Causes

http://bestcbdoil.com/all-natural-pms-treatment/

www.mayoclinic.org/diseases-conditions/premenstrual-syndrome/basics/symptoms/CON-20020003

Treatment

http://bestcbdoil.com/all-natural-pms-treatment/

https://cbdoilreviewer.com/pms-why-hemp-can-help/

http://goop.com/can-cannabis-help-with-pms/

www.hellomd.com/health-wellness/medical-marijuana-may-alleviate-symptoms-associated-with-pms#!

PSORIASIS

Wilkinson, J.D., and Williamson, E.M. (2007, February). "Cannabinoids inhibit human keratinocyte proliferation through a non-CB1/CB2 mechanism and have a potential therapeutic value in the treatment of psoriasis." *Journal of Dermatological Science*, 45(2), 87–92.

www.ncbi.nlm.nih.gov/pubmed/17157480

Symptoms/Causes

www.mayoclinic.org/diseases-conditions/psoriasis/symptoms-causes/dxc-20317579

www.webmd.com/skin-problems-and-treatments/psoriasis/causes#1

www.webmd.com/skin-problems-and-treatments/psoriasis/understanding-psoriasis-basics#1

www.psoriasis.com/what-is-psoriasis

Research

https://echoconnection.org/psoriasis-medical-cannabis-and-cbd-research-overview/

Treatment

https://elixinol.com/blog/hemp-oil-for-psoriasis/

www.massroots.com/learn/topical-cannabis-psoriasis

www.mayoclinic.org/diseases-conditions/psoriasis/diagnosis-treatment/treatment/txc-20317590

www.medicalmarijuana.com/medical-marijuana-treatments-cannabis-uses/cannabinoid-treatment-for-psoriasis

www.royalqueenseeds.com/blog-cbd-can-relieve-psoriasis-by-balancing-immune-systems-response-n423

SCHIZOPHRENIA

The Health Effects of Cannabis and Cannabinoids, Board on Population Health and Public Health Practice; Health and Medicine Division; National Academies of Sciences, Engineering, and Medicine, The National Academies Press, 2017. www.nap.edu/24625

Symptoms/Causes

www.medicalnewstoday.com/articles/36942.php

www.mayoclinic.org/diseases-conditions/schizophrenia/symptoms-causes/dxc-20253198

www.healthyplace.com/thought-disorders/schizophrenia-information/what-is-paranoid-schizophrenia-symptoms-causes-treatments/

Treatment

http://healthland.time.com/2012/05/30/marijuana-compound-treats-schizophrenia-with-few-side-effects-clinical-trial/

http://thehempoilbenefits.com/using-hemp-cbd-oil-for-schizophrenia-and-psychosis

www.mayoclinic.org/diseases-conditions/schizophrenia/diagnosis-treatment/treatment/txc-20253211

http://extract.suntimes.com/extract-news/cannibidiol-cbd-schizophrenia-treatment/

Research

www.civilized.life/articles/cbd-treats-schizophrenia-symptoms/

www.medicalmarijuanainc.com/new-study-cbd-may-help-treat-schizophrenia/

www.projectcbd.org/schizophrenia

www.scielo.br/scielo.php?script=sci_arttext&pid=S0100-879X2006000400001&lng=en&nrm=iso&tlng=en

ULCERATIVE COLITIS

De Filippis D *et al.* "Cannabidiol Reduces Intestinal Inflammation through the Control of Neuroimmune Axis." *PLoS ONE.* 2011;6(12):e28159.

The Health Effects of Cannabis and Cannabinoids, Board on Population Health and Public Health Practice; Health and Medicine Division; National Academies of Sciences, Engineering, and Medicine, The National Academies Press, 2017. www.nap.edu/24625

Overview

www.mayoclinic.org/diseases-conditions/ulcerative-colitis/basics/definition/CON-20043763

www.niddk.nih.gov/health-information/digestive-diseases/ulcerative-colitis

Research

www.ncbi.nlm.nih.gov/pubmed/22163000

Symptoms/Causes

www.crohnsandcolitis.com/ulcerative-colitis/causes?cid=ppc_ppd_ggl_uc_da_ulcerative_
colitis_causes_Exact_64Z186

www.mayoclinic.org/diseases-conditions/ulcerative-colitis/symptoms-causes/dxc-20342757

www.medicalnewstoday.com/articles/163772.php

www.webmd.com/ibd-crohns-disease/ulcerative-colitis/ulcerative-colitis-symptoms

Treatment

www.badgut.org/information-centre/a-z-digestive-topics/medical-marijuana-and-ibd/

www.endoca.com/blog/news/recent-research-showed-cbd-colitis-might-cure/

About the Author

Earl Mindell, RPh, MH, PhD, is a registered pharmacist and college educator. He is also the award-winning author of over twenty best-selling books, including *Earl Mindell's New Vitamin Bible.* Dr. Mindell was inducted into the California Pharmacists Association's Hall of Fame in 2007, and was awarded the President's Citation for Exemplary Service from Bastyr University in 2012. He is on the Board of Directors of the California College of Natural Medicine and serves on the Dean's Professional Advisory Group, School of Pharmacy, Chapman University.

Index

Other Square One Titles of Interest

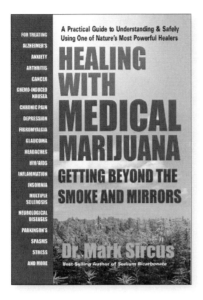

A Practical Guide to Understanding & Safely Using One of Nature's Most Powerful Healers

FOR TREATING
ALZHEIMER'S
ANXIETY
ARTHRITIS
CANCER
CHEMO-INDUCED NAUSEA
CHRONIC PAIN
DEPRESSION
FIBROMYALGIA
GLAUCOMA
HEADACHES
HIV/AIDS
INFLAMMATION
INSOMNIA
MULTIPLE SCLEROSIS
NEUROLOGICAL DISEASES
PARKINSON'S
SPASMS
STRESS
AND MORE

HEALING WITH MEDICAL MARIJUANA
GETTING BEYOND THE SMOKE AND MIRRORS
Dr. Mark Sircus
Best-Selling Author of Sodium Bicarbonate

Healing with Medical Marijuana

Getting Beyond the Smoke and Mirrors

Dr. Mark Sircus

Imagine that there is an effective treatment for dozens of serious ailments—from cancer and Parkinson's disease to headaches and depression. Now imagine that the government is preventing you from using it because it is derived from a controversial herb. Cannabis, more commonly called marijuana, is still looked upon by many people as a social evil; yet, scientific evidence clearly shows that the compounds it contains can reduce, halt, and in many cases, reverse some of our most serious health conditions. In *Healing with Medical Marijuana*, best-selling author and medical researcher Dr. Mark Sircus has written a clear guide to understanding the power of the cannabis plant in combating numerous disorders

While more and more states are now legalizing medical marijuana as a safe and effective treatment method, the controversy continues to block its use for the majority of the population—in spite of the relief it can provide. For those who may be unable to obtain medical marijuana to treat their individual conditions, this book is designed to provide options that can offer the much-needed help they are seeking.

$16.95 US • 192 pages • 6 x 9-inch quality paperback • ISBN 978-0-7570-0441-4

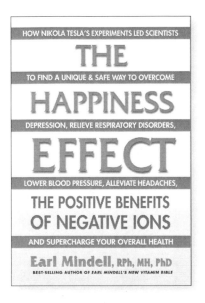

HOW NIKOLA TESLA'S EXPERIMENTS LED SCIENTISTS

THE

TO FIND A UNIQUE & SAFE WAY TO OVERCOME

HAPPINESS

DEPRESSION, RELIEVE RESPIRATORY DISORDERS,

EFFECT

LOWER BLOOD PRESSURE, ALLEVIATE HEADACHES,

THE POSITIVE BENEFITS
OF NEGATIVE IONS

AND SUPERCHARGE YOUR OVERALL HEALTH

Earl Mindell, RPh, MH, PhD
BEST-SELLING AUTHOR OF *EARL MINDELL'S NEW VITAMIN BIBLE*

The Happiness Effect

The Positive Benefits of
Negative Ions

Earl Mindell, RPh, MH, PhD

Imagine a simple force of nature that can provide you with a feeling of well-being, energize you, allow you to sleep better, relieve your allergies, increase your ability to concentrate, and cheer you up. While it may sound too good to be true, it exists, and it's something you cannot get from a bottle of prescription drugs.

The healing power of negative ions has been researched and studied for over a century. The many benefits associated with exposure to these tiny therapeutic chemical elements have been observed and experienced time and time again. Written by best-selling author and researcher Dr. Earl Mindell, *The Happiness Effect* is a complete guide to understanding and using negative ions to achieve a life full of health and happiness.

This book begins with a clear explanation of negative ions— what they are, how they are created, and where they may be commonly found. It goes on to trace the history of man's interest in the nature of electricity, describe the exploratory work that led to a curiosity about these beneficial atoms, and detail the scientific studies that illuminated the effects negative ions have on human behavior and health. Finally, *The Happiness Effect* offers a comprehensive guide to the latest devices that can safely and economically produce negative ions to encourage well-being and happiness.

$14.95 US • 112 pages • 6 x 9-inch quality paperback • ISBN 978-07570-0422-3

What You Must Know About Homeopathic Remedies

A Concise Guide to Understanding and Using Homeopathy

Earl Mindell, RPh, MH, PhD

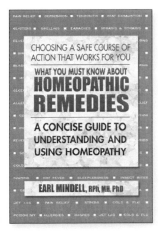

Go to any pharmacy today, and you'll find dozens of homeopathic products that provide relief from a host of health issues—from stress to sinus congestion to jet lag. The fact is, homeopathy has become a widely accepted way of treating many common emotional and physical disorders. In response to the growing interest in this traditional method of healing, best-selling author Dr. Earl Mindell has written a simple and concise guide to understanding and using homeopathic remedies.

$9.95 US • 96 pages • 6 x 9-inch paperback •
ISBN 978-0-7570-0457-5

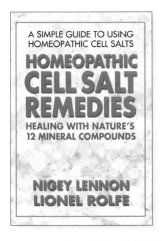

Homeopathic Cell Salt Remedies

Healing with Nature's 12 Mineral Compounds

Nigey Lennon and Lionel Rolfe

Homeopathic Cell Salt Remedies is a simple, comprehensive guide to healing with mineral compounds called cell salts. The book provides full descriptions of the twelve cell salts and discusses how they can be used to treat common conditions.

$12.95 US • 160 pages • 6 x 9-inch paperback •
ISBN 978-0-7570-0250-2

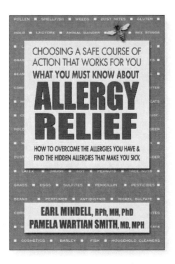

What You Must Know About Allergy Relief

How to Overcome the Allergies You Have & Find the Hidden Allergies That Make You Sick

Earl Mindell, RPh, and
Pamela Wartian Smith, MD

When most people have allergies, they know it. Symptoms come quickly and can range from mild reactions like sneezing and itching to severe, often debilitating effects like anaphylaxis. Millions of others, however, suffer from allergies and don't even know it. Allergies and intolerances are often the hidden culprits that lie at the heart of a number of health conditions. If you are an allergy sufferer or have a recurring health issue that you can't seem to resolve, *What You Must Know About Allergy Relief* is the book for you. Written by a pharmacist and medical doctor, it provides important answers to the most common questions about allergies—what causes them, how they can affect your health, and most important, what you can do to overcome them.

Written in a clear, reader-friendly style, this book is divided into three parts. Part One presents an overview of the causes of allergic conditions as well as their most effective treatment methods—both conventional and alternative. Part Two offers sound advice and practical tips for dealing with asthma, skin conditions, and other allergic reactions both at home and in the workplace. In Part Three, the authors provide a comprehensive guide to anti-allergy medications, supplements, and other treatment options.

Beautifully written, easy to understand, and up-to-date, *What You Must Know About Allergy Relief* offers the tools to identify hidden allergies as well as the means to relieve their symptoms.

$17.95 US • 288 pages • 6 x 9-inch paperback •
ISBN 978-0-7570-0437-7

Apple Cider Vinegar

Nature's Most Versatile and Powerful Remedy

Larry Trivieri, Jr.

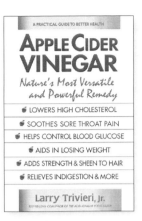

For centuries, apple cider vinegar has been used as a folk remedy to treat a host of health issues, from indigestion and low energy to sore throats and toothaches. As a beauty aid, it can help remove blemishes and add strength and sheen to hair. And that's just the tip of what this amazing elixir can do. Best-selling health author Larry Trivieri, Jr. has written this complete A-to-Z guide that shows how to use apple cider vinegar to prevent and reverse over eighty common health conditions, and to improve and maintain the health and appearance of your hair, skin, teeth, and gums.

$14.95 US • 240 pages • 6 x 9-inch paperback •
ISBN 978-0-7570-0446-9

Turmeric for Your Health

Nature's Most Powerful Anti-Inflammatory

Larry Trivieri, Jr.

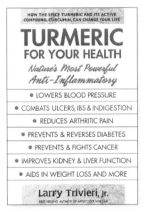

For over 5,000 years, India's Ayurvedic medical practitioners have used turmeric to treat a host of painful and debilitating diseases. Recently, medical researchers in the US have turned their attention to this ancient root and have discovered its effectiveness in lowering blood pressure, reducing arthritis pain, combating gastrointestinal issues, increasing brain function, aiding in weight loss, and much more. *Turmeric for Your Health* is a simple guide to understanding the science behind turmeric's effectiveness. With few if any side effects, turmeric can offer a safe, inexpensive way to enhance your health and well-being.

$15.95 US • 192 pages • 6 x 9-inch paperback •
ISBN 978-0-7570-0452-0

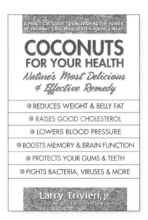

Coconuts for Your Health

Nature's Most Delicious & Effective Remedy

Larry Trivieri, Jr.

Before their introduction to the Standard Western Diet, natives of the South Pacific islands were among the healthiest people in the world. Heart disease and obesity were extremely rare, as were infectious diseases, dementia, and dental issues. Remarkably, the majority of calories consumed by the islanders came from coconuts. Today, medical researchers have rediscovered the many health benefits of this tropical fruit. Coconut has been found to raise good cholesterol, reduce belly fat, boost memory, protect teeth and gums, lower blood pressure, and more. This book focuses on specific concerns from heart disease to high blood pressure to memory loss, and explains how coconut works to combat these issues.

$15.95 US • 192 pages • 6 x 9-inch paperback •
ISBN 978-0-7570-0451-3

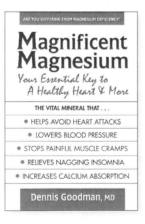

Magnificent Magnesium

Your Essential Key to a Healthy Heart & More

Dennis Goodman, MD

In *Magnificent Magnesium*, world-renowned cardiologist Dr. Dennis Goodman shines a spotlight on magnesium, the mineral that can maximize your heart health without side effects. The author then details magnesium's astounding heart-healthy benefits, along with the additional advantages it provides for other diseases. Finally, he offers clear guidelines on how to select and use this mineral to greatest effect.

$14.95 US • 192 pages • 6 x 9-inch paperback •
ISBN 978-0-7570-0391-2

Dr. Vlassara's A.G.E.-Less Diet

How Chemicals in the Foods We Eat
Promote Disease, Obesity, and Aging
and the Steps We Can Take to Stop It

Helen Vlassara, MD, Sandra Woodruff, MS, RD,
and Gary E. Striker, MD

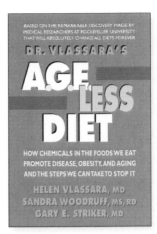

Imagine naturally occurring substances
that are responsible for chronic disease
and accelerated aging. When trying to
discover why diabetes patients were
prone to complications such as heart
disease, Helen Vlassara and her research
team focused on compounds called advanced glycation end
products, or AGEs, which enter the body through the diet.
By lowering your AGE levels, you can reduce the potential
of developing any number of serious disorders and enjoy
greater health.

$16.95 US • 328 pages • 6 x 9-inch paperback •
ISBN 978-0-7570-0420-9

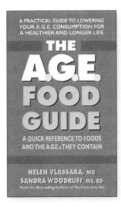

The A.G.E. Food Guide

A Quick Reference to Foods
and the A.G.E.s They Contain

Helen Vlassara, MD, and Sandra Woodruff, MS, RD

All foods contain AGEs—advanced glycation end products—which are naturally
occurring toxins. Numerous studies have
shown that a buildup of AGEs acceler-
ates the body's aging process. Over time,
by increasing oxidation and free radicals,
hardening tissue, and creating chronic inflammation, AGEs
lead to a host of chronic diseases. By knowing how to lower
your AGE consumption, you can lead a longer, healthier life.

$8.95 US • 224 pages • 4 x 7-inch mass paperback •
ISBN 978-0-7570-0429-2

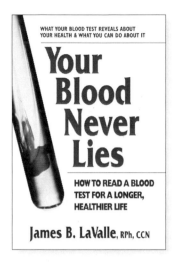

WHAT YOUR BLOOD TEST REVEALS ABOUT
YOUR HEALTH & WHAT YOU CAN DO ABOUT IT

Your Blood Never Lies

HOW TO READ A BLOOD
TEST FOR A LONGER,
HEALTHIER LIFE

James B. LaValle, RPh, CCN

Your Blood Never Lies

How to Read a Blood Test for
a Longer, Healthier Life

James B. LaValle, RPh, CCN

If you're like most people, you probably rely on your doctor to interpret the results of your blood tests, which contain a wealth of information on the state of your health. A blood test can tell you how well your kidneys and liver are functioning, your potential for heart disease and diabetes, the strength of your immune system, the chemical profile of your blood, and many other important facts about the state of your health. And yet, most of us cannot decipher these results ourselves, nor can we even formulate the right questions to ask about them—or we couldn't, until now.

In *Your Blood Never Lies*, best-selling author Dr. James LaValle clears the mystery surrounding blood test results. In simple language, he explains all the information found on a typical lab report—the medical terminology, the numbers and percentages, and the laboratory jargon—and makes it accessible. This means that you will be able to look at your own blood test results and understand the significance of each biological marker being measured. To help you take charge of your health, Dr. LaValle also recommends the most effective standard and complementary treatments for dealing with any problematic findings. Rounding out the book are explanations of lab values that do not appear on the standard blood test, but that should be requested for a more complete picture of your current physiological condition.

Your Blood Never Lies provides the up-to-date information you need to understand your results and take control of your life.

$16.95 US • 368 pages • 6 x 9-inch paperback •
ISBN 978-0-7570-0350-9

Sodium Bicarbonate

Nature's Unique First Aid Remedy

Dr. Mark Sircus

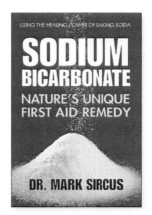

What if there were a natural health-promoting substance that was inexpensive and available at any grocery store? There is. It's called sodium bicarbonate, also known as baking soda. *Sodium Bicarbonate* begins with an overview of baking soda, chronicling its use as a home remedy. Author Mark Sircus then details how this extraordinary substance can alleviate a number of health disorders and suggests the most effective way to use sodium bicarbonate in the treatment of each condition. Let *Sodium Bicarbonate* help you look at baking soda in a whole new way.

$16.95 US • 208 pages • 6 x 9-inch paperback •
ISBN 978-0-7570-0394-3

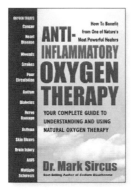

Anti-Inflammatory Oxygen Therapy

Your Complete Guide to Understanding and Using Natural Oxygen Therapy

Dr. Mark Sircus

This groundbreaking book serves as a guide to oxygen therapy, explaining its use in detoxification and as a treatment for disorders such as arthritis and asthma. Special consideration is given to oxygen therapy as a treatment for cancer. Until now, oxygen therapy has been a well-kept secret. In *Anti-Inflammatory Oxygen Therapy*, you'll learn how to use the healing properties of oxygen to change your health for the better.

$15.95 US • 192 pages • 6x 9-inch quality paperback •
ISBN 978-0-7570-0415-5

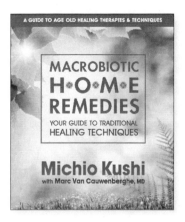
**For more information about our books, visit
our website at www.squareonepublishers.com**